T0207857

THE POCKET GUIDE TO MASTERING YOUR HOLISTIC HEALTH

THE POCKET GUIDE TO MASTERING YOUR HOLISTIC HEALTH

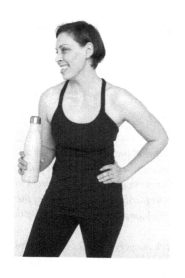

BRIAR MUNRO

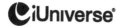

THE POCKET GUIDE TO MASTERING YOUR HOLISTIC HEALTH

iUniverse books may be ordered through booksellers or by contacting:

iUniverse
1663 Liberty Drive
Bloomington, IN 47403
www.iuniverse.com
844-349-9409

Because of the dynamic nature of the Internet, any web addresses or links contained in this book may have changed since publication and may no longer be valid. The views expressed in this work are solely those of the author and do not necessarily reflect the views of the publisher, and the publisher hereby disclaims any responsibility for them.

Any people depicted in stock imagery provided by Getty Images are models, and such images are being used for illustrative purposes only. Certain stock imagery © Getty Images.

ISBN: 978-1-6632-1433-1 (sc)
ISBN: 978-1-6632-1435-5 (hc)
ISBN: 978-1-6632-1434-8 (e)

Print information available on the last page.

iUniverse rev. date: 12/09/2020

DEDICATION

This book is dedicated to my clients. Thank you for allowing me to be part of your health journey, for putting your trust in me and for spending your time and energy implementing my suggestions. It is a pleasure working with you all each and every day.

CONTENTS

PREFACE

When I was 12 years old, I was diagnosed with Legg-Calf-Perthes disease. This is a degeneration of the bones that make up my hip joint. It causes stunted growth in the affected joint, which throws off the alignment of my entire body. This in turn causes a lot of pain and limits my range of motion and the activities I may choose to do.

Now if I were a mathematical or scientific genius, or technical in any way, this may not be a problem. I could work and go through my regular daily routine still in pain but without too much hassle. I, however, am an athlete. I need to move to be happy.

My entire childhood was filled with sports, dancing (many styles), martial arts, swimming, dragon boat, basketball, etc. So getting this news that I had Perthes disease was hard. In fact, I was told that until my first surgery, I should not be walking. The doctors certainly didn't know me! They had no idea that that was the worst message they could have given me. To be honest, my parents and I didn't take their advice. After being diagnosed in 1989, I did my grading for my black belt in tae kwon do in May of 1991 and had my first surgery in September 1991.

When in recovery after that surgery, I had my first experience with physiotherapy. It was at this time that I decided I wanted to work in the health field. I wanted to help people of all ages to be healthy. To me, that could mean healing from an injury, losing weight, exercising safely, eating well, decreasing stress, getting organized or a combination of all these things!

I have spent the past decade utilizing my research and work as a personal trainer, mindset coach and health-care professional to help myself and my clients, and now it's your turn to learn some of my techniques! Some may be new, and some may be reminders to you.

Learning to master your health can be a bit daunting. There are so many aspects that determine how healthy we are, and, I won't lie to you, mastering them all is difficult. In fact, we all go through phases where we focus on a specific area of our health and work really hard at improving it. Maybe we feel that we are on a good path, so we move on to another area. But have we mastered the first one? Or do things slowly slip back to where they once were? Remember the saying "It takes 21 days to build a habit"? In my experience, it can take much longer. Are you ready to get started? If so, then welcome to *The Pocket Guide to Mastering Your Holistic Health*! I want to thank you for deciding to go on this health journey with me.

I would like you to start by taking a moment to thank yourself right now. It is not often that we take time to focus on ourselves. We take care of, or focus our time on, our children, our parents, our spouses, our clients, our work and so forth. How often do you give to yourself? Time and energy just for you? Reading *The Pocket Guide to Mastering Your Holistic Health* and working through the exercises is a fabulous place to start, so congratulations!

Take your time with each section of this book (there is no

rush) and create these new habits in your life so that you no longer need to *think* about them. Eventually they will just happen, like brushing your teeth before leaving the house or eating dinner each day.

I encourage you to get a journal to keep notes about this process. I will be asking you to do some writing exercises. It will be easiest if you get a journal so you have all these writings in one place. I have also left space for you to make notes at the end of each chapter so that you have clear action steps relating to the items you feel you most need to implement into your life. This way, all the information won't become overwhelming.

We will go through your body, both the mental aspects and the physical aspects, and then we will focus on the external environment around you and how you can master this area as well.

I believe that when we focus on the positive rather than the negative, we can create the person we want to be no matter what our past story tells us. We can create our current and future story. My goal is to help you feel comfortable in your own body—and to be happy, healthy and holistic.

ACKNOWLEDGEMENTS

Special thanks to my family. Without your love, support and understanding, my work wouldn't have been possible. I love you and thank you with all my heart.

CHAPTER 1

DETERMINE YOUR DREAM

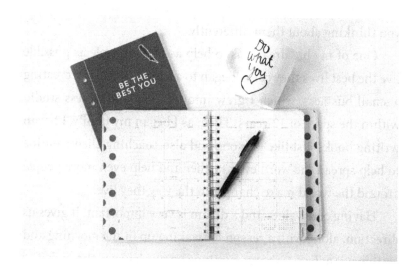

What are your dreams? What would you like to accomplish in life? Big questions, right?! If you already have a dream or even a few of them, then take out a blank piece of paper and write that dream (or those dreams) across the top in big bold letters.

Not sure what your dream is? Let me ask that question in a different way: What makes you happy? What do you want to achieve while you are here on earth? If you were to die tomorrow, what would you want your friends to say about you? What do you want to leave behind? What do you want to be known for?

If you are still not sure about your dream, then let's talk about your core values. Write down what you stand for. What's important to you? What do you believe in? For example, if you choose to purchase organic food, why is that important to you? Why do you drive the car that you do? Or take public transit? Or vaccinate/or not vaccinate your children? If you have a strong core value related to the environment, then perhaps your dream is related to the conservation of the earth. Asking yourself these questions can start to open up what your core values are and get you thinking about them differently.

One of my big dreams is to help as many people as possible live the best lives they can. I began to accomplish this by creating a small business, which I grew into a health and fitness studio within the space of 12 years. Then, as I began my family, I began writing books just like this one and also coaching clients online to help spread the word even farther and help even more people around the world make changes to the way they live.

Having core values and a dream is very important. It gives us direction, along with a reason for waking up in the morning and getting out of bed. So as we continue on our journey through *The Pocket Guide to Mastering Your Holistic Health*, I want you to keep that space clear at the top of your page until it hits you. And it will. When your dream pops into your head, write it down in that top space of your paper. And don't forget to put it in big bold letters so that it is crystal clear.

Importance of Goals

Next, let's talk about why we need goals, how they work for us, how they can move us forward, and how to get motivated to achieve our goals. We will get you started on setting some goals.

Sometimes setting goals can be a bit daunting. There is often a lot of self-talk that stops us from setting goals. We come up with excuses, such as not having enough money or time.

A client I'll call Clare told me that she would love to set a goal of learning a new language so that she could travel one day and have more confidence in herself once she arrived in a foreign country. But she felt she couldn't afford the lessons, let alone the travel. So together we researched and found a free app where she could start learning the language of her choice. We also sourced out one extra job she could take on a few hours per week to begin saving for her trip. We found a starting point for her.

So that leads me to the question, what are goals? Put really simply, they are things we want to do in life. Whether it's to change a light bulb that has been out for months, write a book, go on a trip to Africa or learn a new language, these are all goals. Now you may be thinking that changing a light bulb isn't a goal; it is just an item on a to-do list. Is this true? Well, yes and no. Small items like this one can definitely be on a to-do list for a weekend, but isn't it really just a tiny goal? And if you were to accomplish all the tiny goals on your list, wouldn't it free up more time and mental energy for you to focus on a larger goal? Also, if you saw that you had five goals (big or small) crossed off your list, wouldn't you be more motivated to continue working on the next item on that list?

So, really, goals are anything that you need done, want to do, want to learn or want to try or experience. Goals may entail places you want to go, people you want to spend more time with, and things you want to learn how to do, either for pleasure, for work or for your family. The list of options is really endless!

Over the years, I have done many courses and programs, have read many books and have filled out endless worksheets about goal setting. I am a very goal-oriented person. When I don't have specific things that I am working toward, I feel depressed and confused. I am unsure of what I'm doing or what direction I am going in. In fact, I become very lazy and lethargic, finding it hard to get off the couch! I have found that this is true for a lot of people; they just don't always know that this is what's going on.

As human beings, we need direction. We need a purpose in life. Again, this doesn't have to be a big purpose. I am talking about purpose on a daily basis. Are you working in your home to raise a happy, healthy, productive family? Are you a bank executive working every day to help people get their finances in order? Are you a teacher working with students to help them learn on a daily basis? You chose what you do every day for a reason. What is that reason? I want you to write it down right now. Why did you choose your job? And let's ask a few more questions here while you're thinking: Are you a waitress working every day to give your customers a great meal in a fabulous environment? Do you work in a factory producing items in a timely, functional manner to get them to the clients quickly and efficiently? Do you work for the public transit, getting residents of the city to their locations quickly and safely? Even if you don't love your job, it does have a purpose. What is yours?

Great, now you have remembered or reinforced your purpose.

That's your job. For some people, they may think of a job as nothing more than a job. For others, their job is their way of life, and therefore their purpose may be their motivation to do all sorts of other things in life. If your job is just a job to you, then maybe that is your motivation to learn new skills and try new things outside of work, just for fun. Or maybe the new skills you learn will help you find a job that has more meaning for you. If you truly love what you do day in and day out, do you think of it as a job?

Most of us spend more time working and sleeping than we spend doing anything else in our lifetime. So if you don't enjoy what you are doing right now, or if you have lost your passion for your job, I want you to block off some time for reflection and future planning. Think about why you don't enjoy your job and what aspects of it bother you, then let's work together to go through other parts of your life and find something that you do love!

Many people can sit down and brainstorm a short list of things they want to get done today: do the laundry, grocery shop, take the dog for a walk, answer emails and phone calls, etc. But how many of us write out what we want to achieve by the end of the month, three months down the road, in the next year or five years from now? It gets harder as the length of time gets longer, doesn't it? Many of us are also great at dreaming—huge trips we would love to take, houses we want to have in foreign places, businesses we want to own even—but are we doing anything to work toward those things, or are they just dreams that we think will never come true?

Photo Exercise

What I want you to do right now is take out a photo of the most important person in your life. It can be a physical picture, or it might be one on your phone, iPad or computer. It doesn't matter; just have it in front of you.

When you look directly at the person, how does he or she make you feel? Are you speechless? Are you overwhelmed by love? Are you calm? Do you feel warm inside? Would you do anything for the person? Do you want to be around for a while to see this person progress in his or her life? Would you like to be able to participate in parts of his or her life? Would you like to succeed for this individual?

Take a moment to look at your photo, then say something along the lines of, "You are the most important person to me. I love you. I am taking time away from you right this moment to read *The Pocket Guide to Mastering Your Holistic Health* and learn something new. I am going to do great things. I am going to work hard, make huge strides and be successful. It may take some extra work. I may have to get up early, go to bed later and work twice as hard in between, but I am going to do amazing things, and I am going to make you proud." How does that make you feel? You have just committed yourself to doing something fabulous. You have just made that commitment to change your story, and you have said it to the person who is most important to you. Now what if I were to ask you to make that same commitment to that person directly, in person, to his or her face? Do you think that would make an even greater impact on your commitment to your success? Would you be more likely to change your story?

I personally did this exercise with my husband. After doing the photo exercise, I decided that I really needed to tell him these things. I hadn't voiced my goals to him, nor had I let him know what reaching my goals would mean to me and to our family. Telling him what I was committed to do not only made it a stronger commitment in my mind but also made me accountable to someone else. *And* I had my husband's support on a whole new level.

How about looking yourself in the mirror and saying something along those lines to yourself?! You have the power to take your life in your hands. The power of thought is very strong. If we have any doubt about ourselves and our future, then we will not succeed. But we have the power to change our thought process and make anything possible.

Often we have trouble loving ourselves, so we want to change for other people. It is very important to keep those people in mind, but at the same time you must learn to love yourself. Make these changes for you, so that you create that story for yourself. Become the person you want to be. Let me take you through the steps to realize you have already begun.

Finding Your Peak Attitude

Motivation comes from having what I call a peak attitude. If you were to rate your mood, energy and motivation on a scale of 1 to 10, then level 10 would indicate that you had a peak attitude. So if I were to ask you right now, this very moment, what level you are at, what would you say? Are you feeling like a level 4 today? How about an 8 or a 9? Well, guess what? I bet that we can turn that into a 10 pretty quickly. The thing is that you are already at a 10; you just may not realize it. This is simply because you haven't brought your awareness to it yet. Let's begin taking those next steps to start the awareness journey.

First, I'd like you to write down your three biggest challenges in life. What have you struggled with? What has affected you in a big way? Was it a medical issue, a work struggle, a hard relationship, or struggles within your family perhaps? Please take a moment to write down the three biggest challenges you have had throughout your life. You can jot them down in a bullet list or in small paragraphs, or take this time to truly get them off your chest and let the words flow onto your paper!

All right, now comes the next step. I want you to think about what you have learned from each of these three things and how they have affected your life. Did they help you learn a new skill? Did they open your eyes to how resilient you are? How determined? Did they teach you that you can't help everyone? Maybe you learned how to relate to people differently, or perhaps it showed you how strong you are physically, mentally or emotionally.

Excellent! Now look at that list for a second. Do you realize that you already have overcome the three biggest challenges life has presented you with? You may not be exactly where you want to be with each of them, but then again, have those three things actually stopped you from living? Have you let them? I bet not. I know my three challenges were blips in my life, but they haven't fully stopped me. I have learned from them all, and they have made me who I am today. I can almost guarantee that you have too. You are strong! The things you have struggled with in the past have gotten you to where you are today. You wouldn't be the same person without them.

So think again for a moment about what level you are at. Are you only a level 4 when you have overcome so much? Aren't you really at a level 10? Take a moment now and let that sink in. Do you realize that each and every day you are overcoming obstacles that pop up? Each day you are dealing with situations, big or small, that make you who you are. So finding that peak attitude isn't so hard when it's already there! It is waiting for you to realize that your 10 is within you every day when you wake up. You have the choice to stay at a level 10 throughout your day, or you can choose to let your attitude slip back down. Take advantage of that level 10 each morning and use it to your advantage!

Daily Goals

Next, let's think about some small daily goals that you want to achieve, things such as drinking more water, stretching every day, calling five clients to check in with them, and so forth. I want you to take a cue card and write these goals down in a list with as much detail as possible. So instead of simply "I want to drink more water," write, "I will drink two litres of water per day." See the difference? I have made it an "I will" rather than an "I want," and I was very specific as to the quantity. This is a little mindset trick. I have found that if you constantly tell yourself that you *will* or *are* doing something rather than that you *want* to, then your unconscious mind starts to believe that it's already happening. Then your unconscious will help you to do those things more consistently.

All right, go ahead and make your list now.

Next to your list, you are going to create a chart with the days of the week in the topmost row. This will be your weekly checklist where you can easily mark off when you have accomplished each daily goal. You will be able to look back at the end of the week and see what a fabulous job you have done or, alternatively, where you need to focus more next week.

Daily Goals Chart

	Monday	Tuesday	Wednesday	Thursday	Friday	Saturday	Sunday
Drink two litres of water per day							
Call five clients							
Stretch 10 minutes per day							

Our small daily goals can add some consistency and routine to our lives, which will help us to become better organized and feel more settled so that we can focus on achieving some of our larger goals. This list should *not* be long. Keep it simple so that it is not overwhelming. Also, keeping it on a small card that can be kept in your pocket or purse is ideal. You want to have it with you throughout your day so that you don't forget about your goals and so that you can work on these items throughout your day.

Let's look at some of the larger items next. For this next step, you will need five pieces of paper and an open mind! As you go through this next exercise, try not to worry about how things will be achieved. Just let your mind flow. We will worry about the *how* a little later.

On the top of the first piece of paper, you will write in big, bold letters the word *health* as the title. I want you to brainstorm for a moment all the things you would like to do for your health. These could be short-term goals, such as purchasing a yoga mat to have at home, exercising three days per week, trying five minutes of meditation or reading a health book, or they could be long term, such as running a half-marathon, climbing a mountain, learning to play hockey or exploring your religion or spirituality. Write them down on your health list now.

On your next sheet, write down *education*. On this list you can write down any courses you want to take, any classes you want to sign up for, things you want to learn, books you want to read, etc. My list had things such as learning to knit and learning Italian. I had books for work and pleasure. List them all!

OK, we are really getting someplace now! Bring out your next sheet of paper and, on the top, write down *work*. Now, this list could get long. Try not to write down daily tasks here that need to be done, but think about projects, ideas for new ways of doing things, new ways to pitch ideas, and things you have always wanted to get done but that haven't happened yet. Take a moment to get them all down on paper right now!

Next is our *adventure* category. This one is fun! List all the places you want to travel to and explore, any "crazy" things you want to do such as go caving, skydiving or zip-lining. It could be riding a motorcycle or learning to swim—anything you think is adventurous. Now my adventures may seem like everyday items on someone else's list, or they might seem completely out there. That's all right. For example, on my list I had skydiving, searching for waterfalls, visiting Jamaica and hiking a local trail. Each of us has our own idea of what adventure means, so don't worry about anyone else; just brainstorm your own adventures for now.

Last but not least, on your fifth sheet of paper write *relationships.* This is where we are going to think about all the other people in our lives. Is there anyone with whom you want to connect again, or someone with whom you wish to connect in a different way than you have in the past? Whom do you want to spend time with, and what would you like to do with this person? Is it that you prefer a weekly date night with your spouse? A coffee date with your sister? A girls' night out? One-on-one mini dates with each of your children? Contacting an old friend for a phone conversation? Getting to know a cousin a bit better? Write them all down!

The Big Picture

Wow, that's a lot of lists! I want you to lay them all out in front of you now. Take a look at the big picture for a moment. These are all separate areas of your life. Are your lists balanced? Is one section's list much longer or shorter than the others? This is where you will come to determine if you need to rebalance things. When I first did this, my work list was huge! I had very many things I wanted to do with regard to my career, but the rest of my lists were tiny. This was a real eye-opening moment for me as I realized that I spent way too much time working and not so much time on the other areas of my life. I then went back to my other lists and really thought about what types of things I might want to do. I added those items to those lists. Now my life is much more balanced. Although I still work a lot (because I love what I do), I now spend more time doing other things, and I am much happier as a result. So if your lists seem out of balance, just take note for now. As you go through the next few days, allow your mind to focus on the other areas of your life. Put some thought into what else you may want to do.

Now you have a lot of goals. You may be thinking that some of them are not realistic or achievable and that you shouldn't have put them down. That's all right. *Remember that if you don't set big goals, then you will never achieve big things.* Putting your goals down on your list is your first step toward working toward them. You may have to break down some of the large items on your list into smaller goals. If you want to travel to Greece, you may need to get a brochure as your first step. Then check into the cost of flights and the areas that you want to visit. Then book hotels and travel. Those are all steps that you have to take in order to achieve your big goal of getting to Greece. You may even need to go back farther and set goals for making more money to allow you to purchase your flights. That's all part of the process. Don't think those big goals are out of the question; just break them down and start with the small steps. Choose when you will do those small steps, then write them down either on a to-do list or in your agenda. Make it realistic.

You will get there. When you are sitting in Greece enjoying the spectacular views, you will think back to all the small things you did to get there and you will be so proud of yourself.

Approximately 90 percent of people who read *The Pocket Guide to Mastering Your Holistic Health* will do absolutely nothing when they are finished with the book. Will you be one of those people? Or will you take your lists and your daily goal card and start right now?! I encourage you to post your lists where you can see them each and every day. Put them on a mirror or your front door—someplace that you will pass each day. As you achieve a goal, cross it off your list so that you can visually see what you have done. This will motivate you to keep going.

Also, keep your daily goal card with you at all times, in a pocket or in your purse. As you achieve your daily goals, check them off. At the end of each day, go over your list to make sure you have done each thing. If not, then make sure those things you have left undone get done before you go to bed! At the end of each week, write out your daily goals again on another card for the following week.

Remember, you have already achieved great things in your life. You have overcome the three biggest challenges in your life and have survived! You are at a level 10 each and every day when you wake up, so allow yourself to stay there!

Above all else, remember your *dream*! Your dream will motivate you every day to achieve your goals and work toward your legacy. Go out and get it done!

Notes from Chapter 1

What is my dream? _____

What is my purpose? _____

My three biggest challenges have been:

_____

_____

_____

How I overcame my three biggest challenges:

_____

Other Notes from Chapter 1

_____

_____

_____

_____

Action steps I need to take:

    1)

    2)

    3)

    4)

    5)

CHAPTER 2

THE SOUL

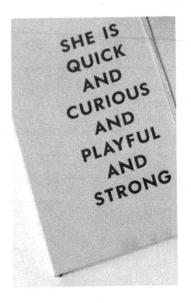

SHE IS
QUICK
AND
CURIOUS
AND
PLAYFUL
AND
STRONG

I often talk to my clients about listening to their bodies. How does your body feel? Is it trying to tell you something? Are you paying attention to it? What will your body allow you to do today? Remember that your body is different every single day based on what foods you ate the day before, how you slept and so forth. Learning how to listen to our bodies is a skill that we all need to learn.

We also need to learn how to listen to our souls. The soul is the true self, who we are deep down without anyone else's ideas imposed upon us. Some people see this as being spiritual; others would say that they are listening for their gut reaction. It's all the same; we may just call it something different.

When I was told that I shouldn't be walking or that fitness was not a good career choice for me because of my hip problems, my soul let me know that those doctors were wrong. I knew where my life would lead me. I can't even imagine what I would be doing today if I had listened to my doctors! Instead I listened to my soul and set out to prove those doctors wrong. To this day, I am still telling doctors that I made the right choice!

Over the years, I have had times when listening to my soul has been hard. In fact, I completely ignored my soul for quite some time. Those were my darker days. It has taken a lot of time and practice, along with some patience, to start listening to my soul again.

We all have strong minds (some of us have overactive minds) that tend to take over for our souls. We have learned "truths" that our minds truly believe, so when we are trying to listen to what our souls are telling us, our minds often jump in with the buts, the what-ifs and the "I don't think ..." comments. Quieting the mind can be tough, but the more you practice, the better you will become at quieting your mind!

The best way to start is by sitting in a quiet space with your eyes closed and taking some deep breaths. Calm your mind. If a thought pops into your mind, just pause, take a deep breath and clear the thought. When you feel relaxed and quiet, ask your soul a specific question.

It could go something like, "Soul, I'm trying to decide if I should take time off work to travel with my family. Is this something that will ignite passion within me, or will I be more stressed upon coming back to work?" Then wait for the response. It may come to you immediately, or it may take a little while. It may come to you in words, pictures or visions of your future.

As you begin to practice listening to your soul, you can use the technique at any time for issues big or small. Are you unsure whether you should eat that chocolate bar? Pause and ask your soul whether your body will be able to handle that type of stress.

What would your world be like if you listened to your soul before doing anything?! Would you be happier? Healthier? More relaxed? Again, it does take some practice as your mind may kick in and say, *Writing a book takes a lot of time, which is something I don't have right now.* But if your soul truly wants something, the universe will help you to achieve it.

We are the creators of our own stories, our own truths. I made the decision that being in a wheelchair was not going to be part of my story. I could have listened to those doctors, but instead my parents and I decided that wasn't going to be my truth. In the time between getting the doctors' suggestions and having my first hip surgery, I earned my black belt in tae kwon do at the age of 12. Yes, I experienced pain and had to do a lot of mental work to overcome the barriers presented by my physical limitations were. But it was my choice, either black belt or wheelchair; those were my options. I created my story.

We all make decisions every single day about how we are going to live our lives. Are we going to work day and night for someone else, or are we going to take some time to create our personal dreams? Perhaps working for someone else allows you the freedom to live out other dreams unrelated to your work. It's your choice. There are no excuses or barriers other than the ones you create for yourself. What are you going to do? What are you going to become? What do *you* want? Take a little more time right now to sit in silence and ask yourself that last question.

Notes from Chapter 2

_____

_____

_____

_____

_____

_____

_____

Action steps:

1)

2)

3)

4)

5)

CHAPTER 3

STRESS

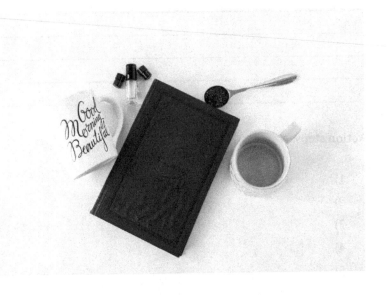

If you are stressed and/or not getting enough sleep (or recovery time), your body will react in many ways. Physical symptoms such as headaches, or even illnesses such as colds or the flu, are the common ones, but there are many other symptoms that occur that we may not realize are caused by stress and sleep. I think that in general we all realize that stress directly correlates to our health, but let's dive into exactly what those correlations are and how they affect us.

What Is Stress?

We think of stress as a bad thing, and in excess amounts it is, but we actually need some amount of stress for our bodies to function. In some cases, stress is a necessary thing. My mentor Paul Chek explains that there are six different types of stress, which all work in a good way and a bad way:

Physical Stress

Physical stress is needed in the form of exercise and movement. When we load our muscles, bones, tendons and ligaments with resistance or impact under gravity, it creates a stress on the body. Exercise at regular intervals is necessary to maintain a good metabolic rate and to remain in good health overall.

The bad effects of exercise can come from not exercising enough but also from overexercise. Not exercising enough can result in weight gain and health issues, whereas overexercising can result in injury and can actually suppress the immune system and keep it from functioning properly. This can lead to respiratory issues, chronic fatigue and a number of other illnesses.

Even poor posture is considered a form of underexercising. Your posture affects your breathing, how your muscles function, your joint health, your circulation and even how well your internal organs are working. If your posture is poor, then your body is out of alignment and unbalanced. The rest of your body's systems will follow.

Chemical Stress

The human body is filled with chemicals that are necessary to our survival. These are natural chemicals that are produced by the body and are necessary to our daily functioning. The production of these chemicals causes stress on the body. This is considered good stress as we need it to function. Take the production of vitamins, minerals and hormones such cortisol and melatonin for example.

The bad chemicals come from our environment and from foods. We are overloaded with chemicals day and night, and we don't even realize it half the time! The human body is not designed to deal with or break down these chemicals; therefore, we store them in our fat cells to keep them away from our internal organs (otherwise we would die!).

Examples of the chemicals we ingest are medical drugs (which are synthetic), and pesticides, herbicides and fungicides, which are used in our farming—not to mention off-gases from furniture, carpets, cars, etc. (We will be talking more about those in our chapter on environment.)

Electromagnetic Stress

The electromagnetic field of the earth is an example of a good stressor. This field helps to control our hormones. An example of how the electromagnetic field affects us is when the weather affects people's joints (especially those with pre-existing joint conditions), muscles and moods. The sun causes fabulous electromagnetic stress for us. In fact, without it we wouldn't be alive!

The sun can also cause bad effects on our bodies. If we do

shift work and sleep all day and are up all night, our system will be totally turned around and very stressed. Also, if we are overexposed to the sun and get sunburned, our bodies will be stressed. Overexposure to radiation from X-rays and ultrasounds, and even low-frequency technology such as microwaves, computers, cell phones and televisions, causes electromagnetic stress and can cause health effects, in turn causing problems for your hormones and even your autonomic nervous system.

Mental Stress

We create positive mental stress when we think positively, set goals, work toward something specific, speak in positive terms and overcome challenges—in short, doing things on our own terms and in our own time as we truly want! This takes work, which puts our system under the good type of stress.

When you think negatively (whether thinking bad thoughts or thinking about the things you don't want), feeling that you need to follow societal norms even if you don't believe in them in order to fit in, you cause yourself negative mental stress. Other examples of negative stress include being rushed, studying too hard and being pushed to do something that you aren't sure of.

Nutritional Stress

Eating clean organic foods, eating a balanced diet to get all forms of nutrients, and eating healthy portion sizes are all examples of good nutritional stress. Your body has to work to digest and metabolize the foods. It also has to work to extract nutrients from the foods. Therefore, this falls under good stress.

When we eat too much food or not enough food, and if we are missing specific nutrients in our diet, we can create negative nutritional stress. Also, if we are eating foods that are processed or filled with chemicals, or foods that we are intolerant of, we are stressing the body in a bad way. The human body isn't designed to do this type of work; it's too much for the body to handle.

Thermal Stress

Our bodies work to keep us at a comfortable or balanced temperature. Our bodies sweat when we are too hot to cool us down and shiver when we are too cold to warm us back up. This is a natural and good stressor, one that keeps our body at a comfortable temperature so that we can function properly internally and externally.

Bad thermal stress comes in the form of anything that burns you or makes you too cold, so much so that your body can't compensate and come to regulate your temperature on its own. This sort of stress occurs when you are amid extreme conditions that you can't keep up with.

The human body reacts to all six of these stressors in the same way, meaning that your body can't distinguish if you are under poor nutritional stress or bad electromagnetic stress, for example. All the types of stress are funnelled together within your body.

Imagine collecting all your stressors together in a sink for a week. They don't compartmentalize; they all mix together. At the end of the week, you have to deal with the full sink load. The higher your levels of stress, the harder it is on your body to deal with.

In fact, stressors as a whole will affect the control systems in your body. All these stressors together activate the autonomic nervous system or ANS. The ANS controls those systems that we don't consciously control ourselves, such as digestion, elimination and blood flow. If your overall stress places too much pressure on your body, then your ability to handle any external stress, such as food and exercise, decreases, and that makes it harder for your body to manage any internal stresses such as illness and disease.

Have you noticed that when you have a lot going on at work or in a relationship, you get colds more frequently? Or maybe you tend to throw your back out? It's your body's way of slowing you down to help you de-stress and get some rest!

The autonomic nervous system is split into two parts: the sympathetic and parasympathetic nervous systems.

The sympathetic nervous system is known as our fight-or-flight system. Fight-or-flight, usually activated under stress, produces elevated heart rate and blood pressure because of a release of stress hormones such as cortisol and adrenaline.

Symptoms of excess stress include the following:

- Digestive issues
- Constipation
- Feeling unrested upon awakening
- Nervousness
- Being jittery
- Increased muscle tension
- Increased inflammatory conditions
- Increased susceptibility to infections
- Anxiety
- Night sweats
- Poor sleep quality (awaking in the middle of the night or not being able to fall asleep)

The parasympathetic nervous system, on the other hand, is known as the rest and digest system. Its jobs are to do the following:

- Facilitate digestion
- Facilitate elimination
- Regulate immune function
- Conserve energy
- Decrease heart rate

The following are signs of the parasympathetic nervous system is at work:

- Incontinence
- Feeling light-headed upon rising
- Mucus secretions
- Depression
- Warm, dry hands
- Increased gag reflex
- Increased allergies
- Decreased respiratory rate
- Decreased perspiration
- Feeling a need to hibernate

When we are stressed continuously or for ongoing periods of time, our energy reserves are being used immediately to deal with the stresses. This means that our sympathetic system is working overtime and our parasympathetic system is being suppressed. This overstimulation can cause chronic fatigue and emotional imbalances. Our goal is to balance these two systems as best we can.

You have to cycle stress and recovery, not just in terms of exercise, but also in terms of life. If you are under a bad form of stress for an hour every day, then you need to find something that releases stress for you and do this for another hour per day to balance yourself out.

There are three stages of stress:

1. Adapting.
2. Adapting but starting to have a hard time handling the stress. At this stage, your body will start to show signs and symptoms of stress.
3. Your body stops handling the stress.

Becoming aware of your stresses early will allow you to make adjustments. In fact, awareness is the first step to change in all areas of your life!

Decreasing Stress

Finding ways to decrease stress is priority number one. This can be really hard for some of us. But look at what is causing the most stress for you. Is it financial, relationship, nutritional or physical stress? Pick the top stressor and start there. When you reduce or eliminate one major stress, the rest of them (or at least the next one on your list) won't seem so bad and will be a little easier to manage or change as you will have more energy reserves after handling one stressor.

Once you have determined your biggest stressor, you need to make a plan for how to go about reducing it or eliminating it. Set a series of small achievable goals to get yourself started. When you achieve one small step, it helps to motivate you to take the next step. Maybe you are wanting to decrease your weight as it is affecting your heart and your best friend wants you to run a marathon with her next year. Think about how you would start training for a marathon when you are not a runner! Maybe you start with walking around the block. First you add distance. Next, you incrementally add some mini runs that are longer in distance, slowly increasing until you feel capable of running the marathon. A side bonus is that you have lost weight and decreased the number of physical and mental stressors on your heart by getting outside for a regular exercise routine.

Another first step is to look for someone who has already overcome the same stressor to help you through it. Having support, encouragement and accountability on your journey is key.

Add a note at the end of this chapter with your top stressor listed at the top of the page. Add the small goals you have set and the small steps that you are going to take in order to help eliminate or reduce that stressor. Start with just one small step to get on the right track! When this stressor is more manageable, add a new page of goals for the next major stress item.

Remember that you need to eat and drink right, move right and think right to help you along this path.

Next, you need to look for activities that you love to help balance your stressful times. Choose from things such as photography, writing, knitting, swimming, walking, reading, scrapbooking, tai chi and foam rolling (discussed in Chapter 8). Anything that won't raise your heart rate will help to decrease your stress and make you feel more balanced.

Let's talk about meditation. Meditation is a great way to decrease stress, but it is super hard for many of us!

Meditation does not need to entail sitting in the lotus position with candles burning (although it could be if this sounds good to you!). If you are like me and have trouble sitting still, why not try a movement meditation as a starting point?

Stand with your feet shoulder width apart. Keep your knees relaxed and your eyes closed. Take a deep breath in as you raise your arms in front of you to chest height, feeling as though you are lifting the air. Exhale slowly as you push your hands down toward the floor. Repeat as slowly as possible, adding a slight knee bend as you push down, straightening your knee as you lift and inhale.

The slower you go, the more in control of your breathing you will be. Focus on your breathing to calm your mind.

Another great movement meditation is to walk the labyrinth. A labyrinth is a circular path made on the floor or sometimes painted on the ground, cut in a field or designed with candles or flowers. Following the path and focusing on your breath will help calm your mind. If you move slowly and at a controlled speed, it may help nurture your soul.

Notes from Chapter 3

My top stressors are as follows:

_____

_____

_____

Other Notes from Chapter 3

_____

_____

_____

Action steps:

1)

2)

3)

4)

5)

CHAPTER 4

YOUR MOUTH = YOUR HEALTH

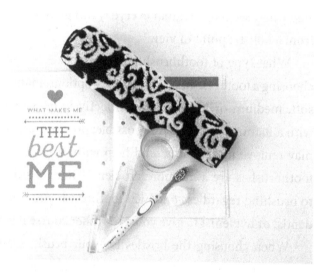

Not many of us realize just how much our mouths mirror our overall health. It has been shown that poor oral health is linked to diseases such as diabetes, respiratory diseases, heart disease, osteoporosis and Alzheimer's disease. It can also cause babies to be born premature or with low birth weight.

Our mouths are full of bacteria, some good and some not so good. Regular brushing and flossing can help keep these bacteria under control. Despite doing this, sometimes bacteria can get out of control and in worst-case scenarios even enter the bloodstream, which is when the real problems arise as this is when other systems can be affected.

Let's look at the health of the mouth, gauging both the external factors and the internal factors:

External: Brushing, Flossing, Using Mouthwash, Going to the Dentist

These may seem like regular everyday things, but let's look at them from a holistic point of view.

What type of toothbrush and toothpaste do you use? When choosing a toothbrush, you have many options: manual or electric; soft, medium or hard bristles. Effectively brushing your teeth with a manual toothbrush is possible; however, an electric brush may remove more plaque and help with gum health as electric toothbrushes are a bit more efficient. There is still a technique to brushing regardless of which toothbrush you use, so ask your dentist or hygienist to give you a refresher course if you need one.

When choosing the bristles for your brush, again, ask your dentist what he or she recommends for you. Each person's mouth, teeth and gums are different, requiring a different strength of bristles.

Toothpaste is one of those things where you have endless choices. It can be a bit overwhelming! Look for a toothpaste that is free of both fluoride and sodium lauryl sulfate. It should also be free of parabens, artificial colors, artificial flavors and artificial sweeteners, and preferably not tested on animals.

Or you can make your own! Yes, that's right. You can easily make your own toothpaste. Here is the recipe:

Toothpaste

Ingredients

2/3 cup baking soda

4 teaspoons fine sea salt (optional), which gives the paste extra
scrubbing power but which can be left out if you find it
too salty

1–2 teaspoons peppermint extract (10–15 drops of food-grade
peppermint essential oil or any other favorite flavor such
as spearmint or orange)

water (enough to achieve the desired consistency)

Directions

Mix ingredients together in a small container, and add water
until your paste reaches your desired consistency.

This is a great recipe for getting rid of bad breath, keeping the
teeth clean and avoiding all the external chemicals of store-bought
brands of toothpaste.

Flossing is super important, not only to remove excess food
particles from between the teeth but also to prevent gum disease.
Flossing with regular floss is your best option for getting in
between the teeth. You can also scrape up and down, cleaning
the sides of your teeth. If you have very sensitive gums, it may be
necessary to start with a gum massager, a soft gum pick or a Water
Pik to help strengthen the gums before moving onto flossing.
Flossing before you brush will allow your brush and toothpaste to
cover more ground and get into all the spaces between your teeth.

Natural mouthwash is the way to go! No more burning,
counting down the seconds until you can spit and spending

frivolous money. Now is the time to start making your own natural, organic mouthwash.

Mouthwash

Ingredients
16 ounces water
1 ounce sea salt
2 drops Living Libations Healthy Gum Drops

Directions

Mix all ingredients in a mason jar and shake before use. I like to use a little shot glass to keep mine from spilling all over the place! Just pour in a bit, swish and spit before brushing and after your mouth-care routine.

Tongue brushing/scraping is also super important! A lot of the bacteria in the human mouth ends up resting on the tongue. By scraping the tongue, it helps to ensure those bacteria are not reintroduced into the saliva and re-ingested by the body. It also helps a great deal with bad breath as the tongue is an escape route for toxins trying to leave the body. You can use a specific tongue scraper, or you might brush your tongue with your toothbrush regularly.

Cleaning the tongue also helps keep the sinuses clear and will reduce the amount of bacteria traveling into the respiratory system.

Teeth-Cleaning Routine

1) Perform the initial rinse with homemade mouthwash.
2) Scrape the tongue.
3) Floss.
4) Brush (brush gums and polish the teeth.
5) Perform the final rinse with homemade mouthwash.

Choosing a dentist is just as important as choosing a doctor. You shouldn't just go to the one closest to you or one whom your friends see. It is important to research your dentist and the practices he or she follows to ensure he or she has values and beliefs similar to yours.

Some dental sealants and composites are high in biphenyl A (BPA). This chemical, which is used to make plastics, can leach into your mouth and saliva as you are being treated and examined. Ask your dentist to use low-BPA products, or look for a holistic dentist in your area.

Most holistic dentists will be concerned with how your mouth and dental products affect your overall health and well-being. They will use mercury-free fillings (as mercury amalgam fillings will release heavy metals into your system, which are toxic); they will use digital radiography rather than regular X-rays to help reduce radiation by up to 80 percent; and they will encourage you to use organic, natural products such as the ones listed above to be made at home!

Internal: Vitamin and Mineral Levels

Many vitamins are important to help maintain the health of your mouth and teeth. These vitamins can be found in all our natural foods!

Vitamin C is shown to be extremely important to oral health. It helps to promote healing of bleeding gums, prevents the formation of plaque around the teeth, prevents gum inflammation and helps promote the formation of connective tissue in the gums. Citrus fruits, bell peppers, broccoli, chili peppers, kiwis, Brussels sprouts, papayas and potatoes have high levels of vitamin C.

Vitamin A, needed in the healing of inflamed gum tissue, can lower the rate of infection and maintains the soft tissue of the gums. Beef, liver, milk, cheese, sweet potatoes, carrots, dark green leafy vegetables, squash, dried apricots, cantaloupe and eggs have high levels of vitamin A.

Vitamin D prevents inflammation and helps the body to absorb calcium (which helps develop and maintain healthy teeth). The best source is sun exposure, but vitamin D can also be found in cheese, milk, mushrooms and fatty fish.

Vitamin E can be used to relieve soreness of the gums. Foods that are high in vitamin E are sunflower seeds, tomato paste, nuts, wheat germ, avocados and turnip greens.

Vitamin B can help prevent toothaches, overall sensitivity in the mouth and receding gums. Food sources include mushrooms, meat, fish, shellfish and eggs.

Iron deficiency can cause your tongue to be inflamed and sores to form in the mouth. Iron can be found in meat, fish, poultry, some nuts, beans, peas, lentils, pumpkinseeds, squash and dark green leafy vegetables.

Notes from Chapter 4

_____

_____

_____

Action steps:

    1)

    2)

    3)

    4)

    5)

CHAPTER 5

SKIN, HAIR, AND NAIL HEALTH

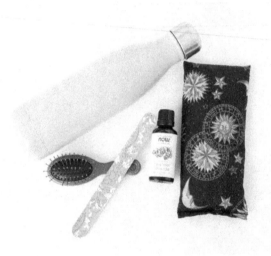

The true way to have healthy skin is to prevent problems! Taking care of your skin from an early age (although it's never too late to start) will truly keep you looking and feeling young.

Here are some easy steps to good skin care:

1) Brush your skin! This helps with lymphatic drainage, reduces cellulite, sloughs off dead skin cells and increases circulation. Add a few drops of lavender essential oil if

you wish to add to your experience. Just put the drops in your hand and rub the dry skin brush in your hand. Then brush in a circular motion from the extremities up toward your heart, avoiding all the sensitive areas. Brush while standing in your shower stall or bathtub before showering or bathing so that the water washes off all those dead skin cells and they go down your drain rather than all over your floor!

2) Avoid long baths and showers as the water will strip your skin of its natural oils. Use warm water rather than hot.

3) Remember, there is no need to wash *all* your skin. Focus on the areas that get smelly: your pits, private areas and feet. The rest of your skin will greatly benefit from not being abused by harsh soaps.

4) Moisturize your skin daily. You may use a natural organic moisturizer or use natural oils such as olive, avocado, coconut, almond or sesame. Let those oils seep into your skin before you get dressed.

5) Keep your beauty products natural and clean. Avoid colors, fragrances, parabens, sulfates and other toxic substances.

6) Drink plenty of water (we will discuss this more, shortly).

7) Sweat regularly, at least 10 minutes per day, to clear out your pores, either through sauna, steam room, hot tub or exercise. More on exercise in Chapter 8.

8) Use a shower filter to decrease the amount of chlorine being absorbed into your body by your skin. The skin is the largest organ in the human body. What it absorbs ends up going through the entire body system. If we are being exposed to toxins daily through our water, it will

be hard for our system to filter that out. So let's use an external filter, which you can find at the hardware store, to decrease the workload on our body's filtration systems.

9) Treat your neck and chest just like your face! These areas are sensitive and are exposed to the same elements as your face.

10) Stop with one glass of wine (or eliminate it altogether). Overdoing alcohol enlarges the blood vessels near the surface of your facial skin.

11) Avoid smoking, tanning salons and sunbathing as they will all age your skin prematurely.

There are many more tips for having great skin, but these are the most important. Really start to read the labels of every product you use on your body, face, head, nails, etc. Remember that your skin is the largest organ in your body and it absorbs everything it comes in contact with. There are already a lot of toxins in the air that we can't avoid, so if we can limit the other toxins that our body is coming into contact with each day, then we will be that much farther ahead on our holistic journey and that much healthier.

Natural Homemade Beauty Products

Face Wash

This is going to sound a bit crazy, but I'm going to ask you to wash your face with oil. Yup, that's right, oil. It is called the oil cleansing method.

Using a mixture of organic oils will help to nourish your skin, replenish moisture and manage the natural oils produced by your skin. Even people with an oily or mixed skin type can benefit. Remember that oil dissolves oil.

Pimples, blackheads, whiteheads, cysts and the like are not the result of oil on the skin. They are the result of hormone imbalances, bacteria, dead skin cells, stresses and/or a combination of all these.

Our skin naturally produces oils because it needs oil. Oil helps to heal, protect and moisturize, and it lubricates the skin to allow it to function properly as the main organ.

Now we also need to remember that drinking water helps to moisturize and lubricate the skin from the inside out, along with helping the skin get rid of toxins. So drink up!

Ingredients to Use for the Oil Cleansing Method

Castor oil, "the oil that heals," has cleansing, healing properties and is an anti-inflammatory.

Extra virgin olive oil or sunflower oil are both calming oils that help the castor oil be absorbed into the skin to eliminate any buildup of dirt in the pores. It sometimes helps to break up the castor oil, which can be thick and sometimes drying. The following are the recommended mixing percentages:

- For oily skin—30 percent castor oil to 70 percent olive oil or sunflower oil
- For balanced skin—20 percent castor oil to 80 percent olive oil or sunflower oil
- For dry skin—10 percent castor oil to 90 percent olive oil or sunflower oil

Mix the oils in a small bottle that has either a pour spout or a hand pump. You may choose to add in five to ten drops of essential oil, such as lavender (for calming the skin) or tea tree (for extra antibacterial effects). Feel free to use more if you prefer more scent.

Pour a quarter-sized drop of oil mixture into your clean hands, and massage your hands together to warm the oils. Gently massage the oil into your skin. Take your time with this and focus on affected areas. The longer you massage, the better the oils will be absorbed into your skin and will grab onto any impurities.

Put a clean washcloth under hot running water. Wring out the cloth, then place it over your face. Allow the cloth to cool. This will gently steam the face, open the pores and allow impurities to come to the surface of your skin.

Gently wipe the cloth over your face to remove the oil. Do not scrub! You are going to repeat the process with the cloth at least once more, and maybe two or three times if you feel the need for extra steaming.

When finished, you will feel relaxed, and your face will feel clean and refreshed and will be very smooth and moisturized.

If you do this in the evening (when deep cleansing should happen), then in the morning you should only need to use a warm face cloth to gently wipe your face and start your day.

If you find that your skin is drying out after a few oil cleanses, then you may need to readjust your percentages of oil or cleanse less frequently.

Shampoo

Ingredients
1 cup water
1 tablespoon baking soda

Directions
Add both ingredients to a squeeze bottle. Shake well before each use.
Section hair and massage into scalp. You may use a fine-tooth comb to work from your scalp down through the hair if you have oilier hair.
Rinse out.

This shampoo will not lather, but by using it you will be avoiding all chemicals and parabens often used in commercial products. And of course you will still get your hair nice and clean!

Conditioner

Ingredients
1 cup water
1 tablespoon apple cider vinegar

Directions
Put into a squeeze bottle and shake well before each use
Use on tips of hair and massage into the ends. Rinse out.

Lemon Exfoliating Body Scrub

Ingredients
1/2 cup sea salt
1 tablespoon olive oil
2 tablespoons lemon juice

Directions
Mix all ingredients in a small bowl.
Apply to hands or feet above the tub or sink so you don't make a mess.
Scrub thoroughly for 2–3 minutes, then rinse briefly with lukewarm water and pat dry.

Body Moisturizer

To make this, mix coconut oil with lavender essential oil (food grade). You can mix it ahead of time in a mason jar. Just fill the jar almost to the top with coconut oil and add in enough drops of lavender oil to scent the mixture gently. Mix with a spoon.

Makeup Remover

The oil cleansing method, discussed earlier, works fabulously for removing makeup while also cleansing your skin. If, however, it is a night when you are doing your oil cleansing method in the mornings, then coconut oil alone will work wonders as a makeup remover! (Also it is great for defrizzing hair and as lip balm.)

Scar/Burn Balm

Mix raw unpasteurized honey with food-grade lavender oil. The amount of oil to use will always be your own preference in terms of scent. The honey can be used on its own, of course, as it holds all the healing properties.

Face Mask

Ingredients
1/3 cup cocoa powder
1/4 cup organic honey
2 tablespoons avocado
3 teaspoons oatmeal powder (blend raw oats until in powder form, or look at your local bulk store for preblended oatmeal powder)

Directions
Mix all ingredients until the mask is consistent.
Apply on the face and gently massage so that the oatmeal can exfoliate.
Leave it on for up to 20 minutes, then rinse with lukewarm water.

Making your own beauty products at home can greatly reduce the amount of chemical ingredients you put onto your skin. Your skin is your largest organ, and it absorbs everything you put on it. Being very conscious of what products you are using is essential. Making our own products may take a bit more time, but it will certainly save you money as you can find a lot of these ingredients at your local grocery store.

Notes from Chapter 5

Homemade recipes to try:

_____

_____

_____

Other Notes from Chapter 5

_____

_____

_____

Action steps:

    1)

    2)

    3)

    4)

    5)

CHAPTER 6

FOOD AND DIGESTION

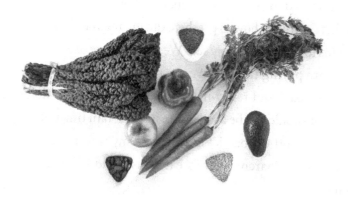

The word *diet* has really been misinterpreted in our society over the years. Diet to me means nutrition, fuel, what foods we are putting into our bodies. I ask my clients all the time how their diet is, and sometimes they'll look at me funny and say, "Diet? I'm not on a diet!" When I ask them this, it is not my intention to imply that they are on a specific diet. Instead, I am talking about their diet in general, their nutrition program.

I think that getting control of one's nutrition is sometimes very difficult. I believe that the way our lives have changed over the years as a society has really made an impact on our nutrition. For instance, we are expected to work 9–12 hours per day, as opposed to the previous average of 8 hours. It is expected that we will be available to be contacted 24 hours per day with all our new technology, and if we don't respond, we are being rude or bad businesspeople. Our children usually are enrolled in three to five different after-school activities so that they may be considered more "well-rounded." We are so busy that we no longer have time to make home-cooked meals or shop for groceries. In fact, our stores had to change to be open 24 hours per day because we couldn't figure out how to get there during regular business hours.

This to me is incredibly sad. We are in a state of chaos, and our bodies are paying the toll. We are relying on caffeine, fast food, and precooked and ready-made meals to sustain us, along with foods that should not be available to us at certain times of the year.

So, right off the bat, let me give you my favorite food saying: "If your grandparents didn't eat it as children, then neither should you!"

Our grandparents were brought up on home-cooked meals that were prepared the same day and often from ingredients that were bought that day, sometimes even directly from the farmers— or even grown in their own gardens. It was part of their daily routine. There were no processed foods to last on the shelves for months at a time. There were no fast food restaurants where people could run in and grab a burger, a sandwich or a salad. Instead, there was a set time for a family dinner each night that everyone made it home by. Kids started their days with real food, rather than sugary processed cereals or Pop-Tarts.

So if you remember one thing, one rule, it should be to eat only things that your grandparents would have eaten. If you keep this thought in the forefront of your mind, then you will really see a change to what you are eating and, as a result of your better diet, a change to a lot of other facets of your health and well-being.

What Does Food Do for Us?

Do you know what a calorie is? What is the definition?

A calorie is a unit of energy. Each calorie we ingest gives us energy to move and breathe, and allows our different systems within our bodies to function properly. Without calories, we would be in serious trouble. In fact, we would not be able to survive. So, again, I have to say that society has turned this word *calorie* against us. Most people think calories are bad for them and they should be eating only the reduced-calorie foods on the shelves at the grocery stores. But this is not the case. Calories are actually important. The problem occurs when we are getting poor-quality calories or too many calories. So let's talk about the quality of our food.

We need to start thinking of our food as fuel for our bodies that allows us to do the things we want to do in life.

Food is often used as a reward, as part of a celebration, or as a way to get together and socialize. This means that we are enjoying our food, which is fantastic, *but* it makes it harder to stop overeating, harder not to overindulge in the sweets and treats. *Why?* Because we are eating unconsciously! Often we are eating while sitting in front of a screen or while working. Rarely are we totally focused on our meals.

Being aware of what we are putting into our systems and why can make all the difference. If we would do this just 80 percent of the time, then our bodies would be able to handle the odd treat, social meal or celebration.

Start tracking! Food journals are a great way just to become *aware* of what you are ingesting. Often we think that we are doing pretty well with our nutrition. Then we start to write it all down, and we realize that we are maybe having too much coffee or that we are allowing ourselves treats after dinner more often than not.

By tracking and becoming aware of what we are eating, we will automatically start to make changes without even having to do much planning!

Organic Food

The difference between organic foods and commercially raised or produced foods is huge! Nutrients are what give our produce and meats their flavor. Organic foods don't look as good, but they taste much better and have many more nutrients.

One of the things commercial farmers do is to put so much salt on the ground that the plants have to suck up huge amounts of water to neutralize the salt if they are to survive. This makes for bigger, lovely-looking produce, but in reality the resulting big fruits and vegetables are nearly empty of nutrients.

You may have read that there is no difference other than cost between organic and commercially raised foods, but you need to look more closely at these articles and studies. Who did the studies, and who paid for those studies to be completed and the articles to be written? There is a great deal of unofficial data, both good and bad, available these days, so you should look at the source before believing what you're reading or hearing.

Here is a good example: The British Soil Association, having analyzed 109 studies on organic and conventionally raised foods, determined that only 27 of these studies were valid comparisons. The rest were done or had been paid for by the companies that produce the chemicals that are spayed onto the crops. Out of the 27 valid studies, almost all of them found that organic foods are significantly better for us.

> Man can only be as healthy as the plants and animals that they eat. The animals can only be as healthy as the plants that they eat and the plants can only be as healthy as the soil they are grown in.
>
> —Unknown

Based on this quotation, we see that it all comes down to the health of the soil. Commercially raised foods are sick because of the chemicals they are raised with. If the food's cells are sick, then we will be sick as well if we eat that food. Whatever the farmer does to the soil affects the end result received by everyone who eats those crops (animals included!).

If our food is no longer natural and is modified, how do you think your body systems will deal with it? The human body is not designed to digest and absorb commercially made chemicals.

Many clients ask me the difference between organic and certified organic. Organic means that there were no sprays, pesticides or chemicals of any kind used to grow those foods. Certified organic also means there were no sprays, pesticides or chemicals used, but it also means that the crops were properly rotated and that the company or farm is being monitored to ensure that it is organic.

There are a lot of farmers out there who farm organically but do not have the Certified Organic title as it can cost a lot of money. If you are purchasing your foods from farmers' markets or straight from butchers, please ask questions. Talk to the farmers and butchers and get lots of information about how they raise their animals, how they grow their crops and if they use crop rotation.

Proper crop rotation means that the farmer will plant dissimilar crops in the same field each year so that the soil can replenish the nutrients that were depleted by the type of crop that was grown the previous year. The soil holds many nutrients, vitamins and minerals that are essential not only to the plant but also to us.

Everything you can find in the human body, you can find in the plant's root system. All our vitamins, minerals, trace minerals and enzymes are in our plants. If we destroy the plant (and its root system along with it), then we will be stripping ourselves of these essential nutrients. That's what's happening right now, unfortunately—and this is why we are seeing a rise in a number of diseases and other health problems.

I will also mention that organic, when applied to a food, means how the food is grown, not how it's packaged or shipped to the consumer. So keep that in mind when you are purchasing products that have traveled to get to you.

How many of us had grandparents or great-grandparents who were overweight? Just 60–100 years ago, there were much fewer overweight people because the food supply wasn't sick and those people were moving a lot more. Doing laundry by hand was a form of exercise. Cooking from scratch was more taxing and therefore meant more movement. There were fewer cars; therefore, people walked more.

Humans exercised more, ate better-quality food and used things like knitting, reading or having tea or dinner with friends as their rest time rather than watching TV, playing video games or going to the movies (all of which, by the way, require the use of too many senses at once and therefore stress us out!).

The food was much less processed, and fewer chemicals were used to grow our foods. Cooking and processing (as is done with breads, cereals, crackers, noodles, etc.) extract nutrients from our foods. Food processing started around the time of World War I in order to make food last longer so it could be shipped to our troops and so that those of us not at war would have food that we could store for longer periods at home.

Vitamins and supplements were introduced around this time as our food was so deficient. In fact, the government made it mandatory for companies to fortify our foods (such as milk and bread) so that we would get enough nutrients from our processed foods. It is fortified because it is dead. We are eating dead food, which in turn is going to kill us!

When we go back through the years and look at cancer, for example, we find that things started getting bad when pesticides and herbicides were introduced to the crops. I'm not saying that all cancer is created by chemicals in and on our foods. Cancer itself is the result of the body's malfunctioning at a cellular level. In fact, we all have cancerous cells; it's just a matter of how well our immune system is handling them. What I'm saying is that all the chemicals we are ingesting are affecting our immune system's strength, and that's partly why so many people are now being affected.

We are in control. We can make decisions about how we spend our money. As a society, if we continue to purchase these sprayed crops, we will continue encouraging the commercial farms to continue using these procedures. If we refuse to purchase these foods and purchase only seasonal organic products from our local farmers, then eventually these commercial farms will change their ways.

Each country has its own laws when it comes to food growth and production. Certain pesticides that have been deemed illegal by one government are still being used in other areas of the world. Foods from all those locations are still allowed to be shipped to different countries though, and they are being sold. We are still ingesting them. But because the foods aren't grown in the countries where they are supposedly illegal, they're still allowed to be sold. We each need to pay attention to the laws in our particular area so that we are aware of what we are ingesting.

What Do Chemicals Do to Our Bodies?

The human body doesn't know how to break down the chemicals that are in our foods because they are foreign substances to us. Our bodies store the chemicals in our fat cells to keep them away from our organs, glands and nervous system. What happens then is that we get fat because our fat cells are at their brink, and our bodies are continuously stressed. In order to reduce this stress, we need to eliminate the chemicals from our bodies.

In order to eliminate the chemicals, you need a healthy detoxification system. And you can't have a functional detoxification system unless you have a functional digestive system. Anyone who's eating cheap, processed or sprayed food is likely to have a digestive system that isn't working. If you are bringing in more toxins from foods than you can release, then your quality of life will decrease.

There are 51 nutrients that have to be in any food in order to satisfy the part of your brain that basically tells you to stop eating. So, what food manufacturers do with processed foods is to selectively remove some nutrients and add in other nutrients. When you eat these modified foods, your stomach sends a message to your brain to say that you haven't gotten all 51 nutrients, so you should keep eating. The problem is that your brain doesn't distinguish what nutrients you are missing, so you often continue to eat the wrong things and, therefore, never have that satisfied, full feeling.

So, yes, certified organic foods are more expensive in most cases, but choosing to spend our money on these foods is really about getting our priorities in order. A good percentage of our income should be going to high-quality foods so that, as a result, we will have to spend less money on health care, prescriptions and other aids to try to make us feel good later.

Protein

Proteins form the major solid matter of our muscles, organs, glands, bones, teeth, skin, nails and hair. Even our blood contains proteins. Without protein, the building and repairing of all bodily tissues and fluids would not be possible.

Where do we find protein? Meats, poultry, dairy, fish and eggs are what we call complete proteins. This means that they have essential amino acids, which are the building blocks of proteins.

We can also find protein in vegetables, grains, legumes, seeds and nuts, but these are not complete proteins. Vegetarian diets must combine two or more of the incomplete proteins to facilitate proper protein synthesis. This is when being vegetarian can be tough for some people as it takes a bit more thought to make sure that each meal and snack has complete proteins so that the consumer of the food is getting his or her essential amino acids, which make the protein usable by the body.

There is a tremendous difference between the quality of protein in the meat from an animal that has been given steroids and the meat from an animal raised on its own accord. The meat from the animal given steroids is lacking certain essential amino acids. When it comes to protein, always go for free-range and organic if possible.

Carbohydrates

Another one of those things that we have been taught is bad for us is carbohydrates. Carbohydrates are our principle source of energy for all body functions. Protein and fats can be converted into energy, but carbohydrates are preferred as they are the only source of energy used by the central nervous system (brain and spinal cord) and the retina of the eye.

Carbohydrates (in combination with protein) form substances that are essential to fighting infection, lubricating joints and maintaining bones, cartilage, tendons, skin and nails.

Carbohydrates are vegetables, fruits, grains, legumes and

beans. You need a wide variety to get a broad range of nutrients. Vegetables are the most nutrient-rich carbs and should be eaten at each meal (including breakfast!). Vegetables should be eaten raw or just lightly cooked to preserve the enzymes and nutrients within them.

When choosing carbs, you should eat mostly lower-glycemic-index carbs such as asparagus, artichoke, avocado, broccoli, cabbage, cauliflower, celery, cucumber, eggplant, greens, lettuce, mushrooms, peppers, tomatoes, okra, onions, spinach, summer squash, zucchini and turnips. These are slower to digest, making you feel full longer, and will slowly raise your blood sugar levels.

Include smaller amounts of higher-glycemic carbs such as fruits, potatoes, yams or carrots, and add even smaller amounts of high-glycemic foods such as bread, rice or pasta as they are very quick to digest and will elevate you blood sugar quickly, giving you the peaks and drops in mood and energy levels.

When having fruit, you should eat the whole fruit. This is best. When you cut a fruit, you lose 50 percent of the nutrients because of the air getting into the fruit. Within one minute of cutting the fruit, even more nutrients are lost. Consume fruit juices in very small quantities, if at all, as they usually have added sugars. If you are going to have fruit juice, then juice the fruit yourself and drink it right away so that you are getting the most nutrients as possible from that juice. Having too many fruits in a day can lead to carbohydrate cravings, so consume no more than four servings of fruit per day.

Lipids (Fats and Oils)

Lipids are vital structural and functional materials to our bodies. They are a very concentrated source of energy and are the building blocks for cell membranes and hormones. They also help to regulate our hormones.

Fats and oils also help in the absorption of vitamins A, D, E and K, which are responsible for healthy nerve conduction within the brain.

When we consume too many altered fats in excess, this can lead to degenerative diseases such as obesity, heart disease, breast cancer and autoimmune and inflammatory disorders. So we have to be careful to have natural sources of fats such as fresh seeds, fresh nuts, legumes, lentils, sprouted grains, green leafy vegetables and fresh cold-water fish. Other examples are flaxseeds, pumpkinseeds, sesame seeds, sunflower seeds, avocado, aloe vera juice, meats, dairy and oils.

Just a side note about oils: they should be stored only in dark glass bottles and kept in a cool place. Canola oil is highly processed and has trans fats (which are man-made), so it's not a good choice as trans fats are hard to digest. Also, the smoke point matters when cooking with oils. The more refined an oil, the higher the smoke point. What is the smoke point? It is the temperature at which an oil starts to burn and smoke. If an oil is overheated, it can lose its nutritional benefits and create harmful free radicals. For example, flaxseed oil and walnut oil should only be used for cooking at very low temperatures as these oils will go rancid when exposed to heat. The best oils/fats to cook with are natural organic butter or coconut butter/oil as these can be used in your body as an immediate form of energy.

Fats such as margarines, shortenings, salad dressings and snack foods all have hydrogenated fats in them. These types of fats raise your LDL cholesterol (the bad kind) and lower your HDL cholesterol (the good kind). This can lead to development of heart disease.

Hydration

We have all been told how important water is to keeping our systems working efficiently. We have heard over and over again that we should be drinking six to eight cups of water per day and that, if we are exercising, we need more. Well, hold onto your seats for a moment, because you really should be drinking half your body weight (in pounds) in ounces of water per day!

For example, a 200-pound person needs to drink 100 ounces of water each day (12.5 cups/day). A 175-pound person needs 87.5 ounces of water each day. So for the 175-pound person, that means just over nine cups of water (if he or she isn't exercising).

When talking about that much water per day, the question I get most often is, "What counts as water? Can I have herbal tea? Watered-down juice? Perrier water?" My answer is really simple: Nothing substitutes for water, not tea, not juice, not beer—nothing!

Always choose top-selling brands such as Evian and Fiji because they sell the fastest and therefore the water has the least exposure to the plastic bottles it's sold in. Or purchase either a filtered bottle to keep in your fridge or a filter for your tap. If possible, buy water in glass bottles instead. Store your water in glass or a BPA-free bottle.

The healthiest waters are the hardest with a hardness factor of 170 mg/L or more. Water that has been subjected to the process of reverse osmosis, which everyone is talking about lately, is actually too soft. Reverse osmosis means that all the bad nutrients have been taken out, but so have the good nutrients and minerals. A filtration system on your tap is a good idea as it filters out the bad stuff but leaves in all the nutrients that you need. In fact, a filtration system on all your taps, shower heads and so forth would be smart as your skin absorbs the chlorine, fluoride and other toxins.

Also, for people who don't have sodium issues, adding a pinch or two of quality sea salt to your drinking water is recommended to replace any electrolytes that have been lost. This is important specifically if you are exercising. It is even more important if you are someone who sweats easily. The sea salt also helps to harden otherwise good but soft waters and makes them much more absorbable by your system.

Urinating seven to nine times per day is normal! So don't be worried if the addition of more water is making you have to urinate more often.

Coffee

Coffee directly affects the adrenal glands, which do many things. One of their functions is to control hormones. Women's hormones are more fragile and go through enough ups and downs throughout a day, but having coffee will make it even harder for these hormones to remain at stable levels. When our adrenal glands are stressed by coffee, it makes us more susceptible to illnesses, stretch marks and much more! Also, coffee is a diuretic and therefore wipes out the water in the system. If you are going to have coffee, drink a full glass of water first to compensate for the coffee you are about to drink. In fact, have your water and then re-evaluate if you even still want your coffee. Often you will find that your body was just craving liquid, not coffee specifically.

So let's talk about ways to slowly get you to choose better coffee options and eventually get off coffee altogether. Your first step in making the coffee switch is to move to drinking only organic coffee. Not only is it better for you as it has fewer chemicals (coffee bean crops have one of the highest percentage of chemicals sprayed on them), but also it tastes way better!

Secondly, know that drip coffee is your worst option. The higher the drip time, the higher the caffeine content. Move to an espresso or Americano (espresso with water added) as it is cleaner and has less caffeine.

Adding unsalted grass-fed butter, MCT oil (derived from coconut oil) or nut oils (hazelnut or roasted pumpkinseed oil) to your coffee will slow down the absorption of caffeine and help your body to see coffee as a food to digest. You will also have less of a crash later in the day. You can experiment with flavors by mixing different fats for taste. But it is suggested to begin slowly by adding only a teaspoon of these fats to your cup of coffee. Then slowly increase this amount to a tablespoon. Maybe start with a mix of grass-fed butter and MCT oil, just as an example.

Never have coffee on an empty stomach as it stimulates

ulcers. Never have coffee after 3 p.m.! If you do, you may have trouble falling asleep or may wake up through the night because the caffeine prevents your body from going into its full REM sleep cycle.

Sugar

Sugar is another thing that is very difficult for most people to cut out of their diets as it is addicting. Any white sugar or processed sugars are bad for the human body because they suppress our white blood cells from functioning properly. These are the blood cells that control the immune system. So it's important for us to get rid of processed sugars.

Your next step is to look at any sugars that you add to your foods. If you are baking, you need to find replacements for sugar. Stevia is the best as it is a natural herb and doesn't change one's blood sugar level. Agave nectar, brown rice syrup and honey are better than sugar but are still highly processed. Having raw, unfiltered and unpasteurized honey is a good choice. Or try manuka honey (made in Australia and New Zealand by bees that pollinate the native manuka bush) as it has antibacterial effects above and beyond regular honey and can protect against damage caused by bacteria. If you tend to add sugar to your coffee, try other options, such as first switching from white sugar to brown sugar. The next step is to go from brown sugar to raw sugar, then to Stevia. Then slowly decrease the amount you are using until you don't need it at all!

A single teaspoon of sugar affects the immune system by decreasing its ability to function by 50 percent for four hours!

After those four hours, the immune system is still not functioning up to speed and therefore is still being compromised—from just one teaspoon of sugar! No wonder there is such a high incidence of colds and flu going around!

Flours and Gluten

White and processed flours raise your blood sugars and affect your mood and energy level. Cut them out! If you are going to use flours in your diet, then choose the least-processed versions: whole wheat, sprouted grains or almond flour.

Many people are finding that they are sensitive to gluten. In fact, about 85 percent of our population has a gluten sensitivity but aren't aware of it yet. Gluten is the protein molecule in most grains. This includes wheat, rye and barley, to name a few. The problem in our society today is that many of us are eating way too many grains, and most of the grains that are being chosen are highly processed. Although it is tough to do so, most of the people who minimize or eliminate processed grains find that they feel much better. If you are going to eat grains, please stick to whole grains added to salads, stir-fries, yogourt, fruit, etc.

You may not think that you are intolerant because you eat wheat and grains all the time and you feel fine. But you may be having a reaction at some level. Often people get a bit of a punch in the lower abdomen as gluten swells the intestines. Sometimes people experience acne, rashes, bumps on the upper arms, etc. You can find out if you are sensitive to gluten through a blood test, but the easiest way is to completely eliminate all grains, except the ones listed below as tolerable, from your diet for three weeks. If you feel better, then you are most likely gluten intolerant.

People with gluten intolerances should avoid barley, brown flour, white flour, Kamut, semolina, wheat, udon, couscous, graham flour, rye, spelt, teff and pastas (except corn pasta or rice pasta).

Foods that are tolerable are amaranth, buckwheat, chickpea flour, bean noodles, rice, tapioca, taro, arrowroot, corn, millet, potato flour, sorghum flour, urad (peas) flour and yam flour.

If you find that you are intolerant to gluten but have been eating it, you should eliminate it for sure, but also eliminate dairy from your diet for three months as the damage to your intestines will make it difficult for you to digest dairy. You can then slowly reintroduce dairy to your diet and see how you feel. If you reintroduce dairy too quickly, then you will have reactions because dairy is a bit tough for your digestive system to break down.

If you are allergic to or intolerant of dairy, other options include coconut milk, almond milk and hazelnut milk. Processed soy products aren't great, because they have a very high content of estrogen. We need to be careful of the amount of estrogen we ingest because too much estrogen can lead to different cancers. These days, soy is added to a lot of our foods. Soy has been shown to be the reason our youth are hitting puberty at such a young age.

Digestion and Elimination

If you are eating a lot of processed foods, then focus on reducing these as one of your first steps. Start shopping around the perimeters of the grocery store only. This is where you will find all your produce, meats, poultry and dairy. The majority of your foods and meals should come from these areas of the store. The inner aisles are where all the processed foods are.

The longer a food is able to last on the shelf, the worse it is for you. Nothing that you should be eating should last more than a week or so. If it lasts a month or a year, then it surely has a lot of chemicals in it or the food processors have had to kill all the enzymes.

Most people eat way too fast. You can cripple the digestive system easily by eating at high speeds. There's an old Tibetan saying: "Drink your food and chew your water." This means that you should chew your food until it's a liquid and that when you drink a liquid, you shouldn't just gulp it down. You should move it around your mouth as though it were food because that mixes saliva with the water. The saliva, which carries the energy from the spleen, enlivens the water so it actually will have a therapeutic effect on the body. If you just gulp a lot of water straight into your stomach, it can be very stressful to your body.

You should always sit down to eat so that your blood can go to your digestive system to help it out. Also, you should never do anything stressful when you are eating. So, talking about happy subjects, listening to calming music and not watching the news are always helpful. Your eyes are linked to your digestive system by reflexes, so if you are doing other things while eating, you are drawing energy away from your stomach.

A healthy digestive system could take 16–20 hours to fully digest foods and pass them through your system.

The average person has a bowel movement once every two to three days. However, you should be passing about twelve inches of well-formed, non-foul-smelling, fluffy, easy-to-pass, light brown, earthy-smelling stool per day if you've got a healthy digestive system. That could be all at once or over a few bowel movements throughout the day.

If you're eating more protein than you can process, it produces urea as a by-product, which is not a pleasant smell at all. Your perspiration will also develop a strong pungent odor. If you are healthy and your body is sweating, it won't have any smelly toxins to release. It will just be sweating water!

Serving Sizes

Knowing how *much* food to eat can be a bit tricky. However, we have a pretty good rule of thumb that is proportional for each individual. We are going to use your hand size to help us determine how much of each type of food you should be consuming at each meal. If you are a taller, bigger-boned person, then your hand size will be a bit larger and you will be allowed to consume a bit more food then someone who is petite all over.

- Protein—1 serving = the palm of your flat hand
- Vegetables—1 serving = the size of your fist
- Carbs—1 serving = the size of your cupped hand
- Fats (healthy fats)= the size of your thumb

You may be asking, "So, where do fruits fit into this?" Well, we actually put high-glycemic-index fruits into the carb category and low-glycemic fruits into the same category as vegetables.

Fats can also be a bit tricky to figure out. Healthy fats that are measurable by comparing them with the size of your thumb include items such as the oils that we cook with or use as salad dressing and nuts. If you are looking at a food such as avocado, which is a great healthy fat, know that it is also considered to be a fruit, so having a serving the size of your fist would be fine as the avocado is providing nutrients from two food groups.

Hopefully this helps you to figure out your portion sizes for foods easily, even if you are out at a restaurant. This is often where people will overeat as their plates are much larger than they need to be and their carb portions (and sometimes proteins) are often much larger serving sizes than an individual needs in one sitting.

Other Tips

- Avoid anything white (and foods that are made with the "white devils": white flour, white sugar, table salt and processed dairy).

- If you must use dairy products and you can't acquire raw dairy, always opt for certified organic as your first choice. Also, for those who are sensitive to milk (lactose), try full-fat cream, which is low in lactose and high in fat (and therefore more easily digestible). You can also try a high-quality yogourt, in which the lactose is predigested.

- If you need to season foods and water, do so with 100 percent unprocessed sea salt. The best is Celtic, followed by sea salt from New Zealand because heavy metal toxicity is lowest there. Or better yet, use only fresh herbs as your flavoring.

- Eating breakfast is super important! Try to eat something (even if it's small) within 30 minutes of awaking. This will jump-start your metabolism and start your body burning calories more efficiently, which will continue for the remainder of the day.

- Never skip a meal! Each time you do so, you increase the fat-storing enzymes in your body. Basically, your body needs food to release as energy, and when you don't eat, your body stores things as fat to be released slowly later so that you don't die!

- Use snacks when needed, but don't force them if you are still full from your last meal.

- Try rotating foods and drinks on a four-day cycle. If you eat the same things every day, it overstimulates your immune system and may cause you to start being sensitive to the foods that you love.

- Follow the 80/20 rule. If you live right 80 percent of the time, you can absorb the other 20 percent!

Notes from Chapter 6

_____

_____

_____

Action steps:

1)

2)

3)

4)

5)

CHAPTER 7

SLEEP

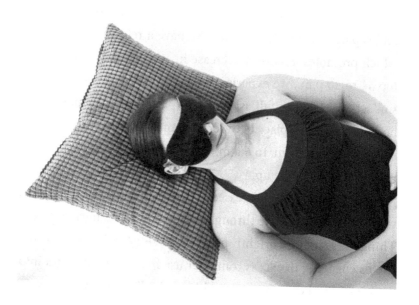

The human body follows the circadian rhythms of the earth, which are made up of the sun–moon cycles. This means that we are in sync with the light–dark cycles of the earth. So whether you are getting four hours or 12 hours of sleep won't matter unless you are sleeping at the right time of the night. Going to bed at 1 a.m. and waking up at 9 a.m. won't do you much good as your body won't feel rested since you weren't sleeping during the proper circadian rhythm times.

Whenever light stimulates your skin or eyes, your brain and hormonal system think that it's morning. In response to the light, your body releases cortisol, which is the activating hormone that is released in response to stress. Light is considered to be an electromagnetic stress. The release of cortisol prepares you to wake up and get moving.

Our natural cycle in relation to the sun and our cortisol levels would have us awaking at 6 a.m. with accelerated activity between 6 a.m. and noon as our levels peak around 9 a.m. Between noon and 6 p.m., our levels drop and we have a release of melatonin, which promotes a natural decrease in activity and energy. From 6 p.m. to 10 p.m., we experience a natural winding down as the sun sets. We should fall asleep by 10 p.m. Physical repair of the body mostly takes place between 10 p.m. and 2 a.m. while we are sleeping. From 2 a.m. to 6 a.m., our system is focused on mental repair, until we wake up.

If we are extremely stressed or stressed in the negative ways, we have cortisol release throughout the day above normal levels. Things like having a brightly lit house, having the TV on, working late or engaging in excess computer use in the evenings and into the night can keep your cortisol levels high, which will prevent your body from releasing melatonin, which is our natural sleep aid. Cortisol can take hours to clear from the bloodstream. Therefore, if you have excess cortisol, you will have trouble falling asleep or else your sleep will be disrupted, which in turn will interrupt your repair cycles.

Excess production of cortisol can result in adrenal fatigue. Adrenal fatigue can present itself in many different ways, but the most common are twitching eyes, chronic fatigue, viral infections, bacterial and fungal infections, and headaches, to name a few. If your adrenal glands are fatigued, it is very important not only to reduce as much stress to your body as possible but also to follow your circadian rhythms by going to bed on time.

The main way to disrupt your sleep once you have gotten to sleep is to use stimulants of different types throughout the day. Caffeine, sugar and tobacco are the most common stimulants. Caffeine has a half-life of six hours. A regular drip coffee has 300 mg of caffeine. If you drink coffee at 3 p.m., then at 9 p.m. you will still have 150 mg of caffeine in your system. Six hours later, at 3 a.m. (during your mental repair time), you will have 75 mg still in your system. This caffeine stimulates your adrenal glands and produces cortisol, which is meant to wake you up!

Eating sugars will increase your blood sugar levels. Blood sugar levels increase after any meal and cause the release of insulin to break down the blood sugar and store it. If you eat high-glycemic foods, the result is an overcompensation response of insulin, which in turn leads to low blood sugar. Low blood sugar can be a major stressor to your body. This then results in cravings for more sugar or caffeine. The cycle keeps your cortisol levels elevated, which keeps your body from winding down for sleep. It's a vicious cycle!

Electromagnetic pollution is a major cause of interrupted sleep. Keep electronic devices out of your bedroom. You are already getting low levels of electromagnetic stress from the power lines, the electrical circuits in your walls, the lights on the ceiling and so forth. You don't need any more stresses.

Setting an evening routine can really help when it comes to the quality of your sleep. Spend an hour before bed calming down with low lights. Drink hot water with lemon to cleanse your system, read a relaxing book and do some stretches. This tells your body it's time to prepare for sleep.

Also making sure your room is pitch-black and removing all electronics (electric blankets, clocks, lights, cell phones, iPads, etc.) from your room will help your sensory receptors to relax. Adding blackout curtains that don't allow any light through from the street or the moon is a great idea.

Also remember never to do strenuous exercise or drink alcohol late at night, and avoid caffeine after 3 p.m., as these are all stimulants.

Notes from Chapter 7

_____

_____

_____

Action steps:

1)

2)

3)

4)

5)

CHAPTER 8

MOVEMENT AND EXERCISE

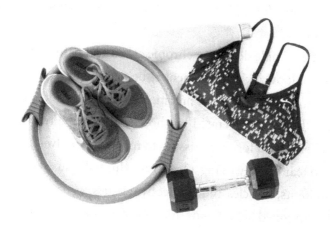

W hen it comes to movement and exercise, it is important to understand how the body moves and how everything is integrated together. The human body works as a pump system. If we are functioning "properly" on account of good stresses, good amounts of movement, good foods and a proper amount of recovery time, then our system is adequately pumping our fluids through our bodies. This way, our muscles contract, forcing water, blood and oxygen through our bodies for optimal function.

If you are not moving enough, you will start to get symptoms such as a low energy level because not enough nutrients are being transported throughout your body. Also, you will have difficulty managing your blood sugar levels. Muscles consume blood sugar at a natural pace. Without enough movement, your body cannot eliminate toxins effectively and cannot absorb the nutrients it needs.

As we age, our metabolism slows down. Most of us continue to eat the same foods in the same amounts that we did when we were younger, without adding (or in fact decreasing) to the amount of exercise we are doing. The end result if this issue is not addressed is weight gain.

A lot of people deal with chronic aches and pains. These are often a result of lack of movement as being sedentary starves the muscles and joints of water, nutrition and oxygen and makes it hard for the waste generated by those tissues to be removed. It also makes it hard for those tissues to repair themselves after the wear and tear of daily living. Over time, this will cause aches and pains to joints, muscles and connective tissues.

As mentioned before, movement helps to deliver nutrients to the body, but it also helps us to eliminate waste. If we aren't moving, then our digestive system can't dispose of waste effectively, which leads to constipation. With constipation comes an increased risk of disease on account of a backup of waste products in our bodies and a lack of nutrient absorption.

Without enough movement, the nutrients that are ingested do not get to the nervous system or the hormonal systems, which are composed of the organs and glands that are responsible for maintaining emotional balance. This can cause mood swings and emotional imbalance.

Next let's discuss the heart. The heart is not meant to pump blood all by itself. With proper movement, the body's muscles help to circulate the blood. This decreases stress to the heart and allows the rest of the cardiovascular system to function properly.

When looking at an exercise program, people tend to migrate toward things they are good at. If squats come easily to you, then you are more likely to add squats to your workout. If you are naturally flexible, then you probably don't mind stretching. The problem is that the things we don't enjoy are the things we need the most.

Let's break it down a bit into a few categories here:

Warm-Ups

Warming up before exercise is extremely important in order to make sure your body is prepared for what you are about to ask it to do within your exercise session. Getting the blood flowing quickly through all the joints and waking up the muscles and fascia takes only a few extra minutes of your time, but it can be a lifesaver in the form of preventing injuries!

Dynamic movements are best done before your workouts. Think about moving through a range of motion in each major joint.

- Arm swings, forward and back, as well as opening the arms and crossing them over the chest
- Shoulder rolls, forward and backward
- Torso twists
  Stand with feet shoulder width apart, knees bent and tummy held in. Then gently twist the upper body from side to side while keeping your hips still.

- Hip circles
  Keeping the torso still, circle the hips as though using a hula hoop!
- Leg swings, forward and back, as well as across the body and opening to the sides (use your tummy muscles to help you balance on your standing leg, with the standing leg slightly bent)
- Ankle circles
- Wrist circles

Do each of these range-of-motion exercises five to ten times. It should take only about four to five minutes.

Even going for a five-minute walk around the block is a great warm-up. Just make sure you are also moving any other major joints that you will be using during that day's workout.

Movement Patterns

Back in the caveman era, there were seven key movement patterns that people needed to be able to do in order to survive. These patterns are squatting, bending, lunging, pushing, pulling, twisting and walking (gait patterns). Nowadays, we need do these things in order to perform daily tasks and remain injury-free.

If any of these movement patterns are compromised, then we will have restricted movement and, in most cases, will be setting ourselves up for injuries.

Many adults lack balance and motor skills because as babies they were rushed through, or else forced to skip, the tummy crawling and kneeling crawling stages and were encouraged to walk too soon. This means that the inner and outer muscles of the core never learned to work together properly in unison. These people may even now have trouble with the primal movement patterns as a result. Ball exercises are best to reteach the inner-outer muscles to function better as one unit and to gain better motor skills, balance and core stability.

Here are a few examples of ball exercises:

- Ball bouncing
  Sit on an exercise ball with your feet flat on the floor about hip width apart or wider. Press your feet into the floor and start to bounce. Start small and slowly increase your height. Make sure to maintain control!

- Ball bridging
  Lie on the floor on your back with your heels on the exercise ball and your legs straight. Have your feet shoulder width apart and your toes pointed up to the ceiling. Turn your palms upward on the floor to help relax your upper body (the wider your arms, the more stability they will give you). Press your heels into the ball and slowly lift your hips off the floor into a bridge-like position. Return to a resting position your with hips on the floor. When you have gained stability here, slowly bring your arms closer to your hips or even up in the air to increase the level of difficulty.

- Alternate arm/leg Superman on ball
  Slowly place your tummy on the exercise ball with your hands and feet touching the floor. Start by lifting one

arm off the floor and then putting it back down. Then do the same with the other side. Then try lifting one foot off the floor and lowering it. Then do the other side. Just get a sense of your stability and balance here. Think about your tummy holding in and the lifting limb reaching away from you. When that feels good, you can move on to lifting one arm and the opposite leg at the same time. The slower you go, the better it will be as it will challenge your balance and core muscles a little bit more.

Core

We talk a lot about core during workouts, especially in Pilates and weight lifting sessions. But did you know that the core includes the entire torso, including your internal organs? The core is our foundation for movement as the extremities rely on the core for stabilization and force production. Joseph Pilates had a saying: "Strengthen the core and the rest will follow."

When we exercise correctly, our internal organs are mobilized, keeping them from adhering together, which improves fluid movement and helps bowel function. The rib cage and outer abdominal muscles help protect the organs.

All movement (but specifically movement of the core) helps to circulate blood and lymphatic fluid through the body.

We have an inner unit and an outer unit of the core. The inner unit is almost like a box within the center of the body. It is made up of the multifidus—deep muscles running along the spine (the back of your box), including the pelvic floor, which runs along the base of your pelvis (the bottom of your box); the transverse abdominis, which runs along the lower part of your stomach and acts like a belt (the front of your box); and the diaphragm (the top of your box). These all function together as a unit to stiffen the spine, rib cage and pelvic girdle so that your extremities may have a stable foundation. If your inner unit stops functioning properly, you can't stabilize properly, and when you go to move your limbs, you are more likely to be injured (specifically your lower back).

Because all these parts of the inner unit work together, when you strengthen one of them, the rest follow—and gain some residual strength too! One of the best types of exercises to strengthen your inner unit are Kegel exercises (or pelvic floor exercises). These are subtle, which means it can be tricky to know if you are doing them correctly. But it also means that you can do Kegels whenever you want and no one will ever know!

The easiest way to know if you are doing Kegel exercises correctly, or to recognize the feeling of the contraction and relaxation of the pelvic floor muscles, is to practice while urinating. Start and stop the flow of urine frequently as you are going. It is your pelvic floor muscles contracting to stop the flow. Relaxing these muscles begins the flow. When you recognize that feeling, then you can practice doing Kegel exercises when sitting in a chair, when lying on your floor or while driving—any time at all!

The organs of the body use the same pain-sensitive nerves that the muscles around them use. So if an organ is in pain, the brain can't tell if it's the muscle or the organ. Therefore, the brain will actually tell the body that everything in that area is hurting. An example of this is when you get lower back pain during your menstrual cycle or you get chest and arm pain during a heart attack. Pain always causes weakening of the muscles!

Anything that causes inflammation to the lower abdominal area (foods to which you are intolerant, your menstrual cycle, constipation, stress, alcohol, preservatives, colorings, medical drugs) will shut down the inner unit, making the muscles weaker and unresponsive.

Therefore, if you have any inflammation in your lower abdominal area, you should take extra care when training in order to help prevent injury. In fact, some days it may be best to rest rather than to push through a workout. Or use it as an active recovery day!

The outer unit of the core consists of the large muscles that move the body. These muscles, which usually cross multiple joints and are easily seen on the outside the body, are the rectus abdominis (also known by some as the "six-pack"), the oblique abdominals (which run along the side of your trunk, forming your waistline) and the erector spinae (the outer muscles running along either side of your spine).

In order to stand upright and move with balance, you need these large muscles to work together, creating balance from the front to the back of your body. You also need to have a strong inner unit. This is very important when it comes to your workouts as often you may have a favorite body part to train. Keep in mind this need for balance between the front and back of the body, especially when it comes to training the core. Don't forget to work your extensor muscles and your entire posterior chain (the backside of your body!). You can do this with a Superman exercise, for example.

Lie on your tummy with arms outstretched above your head. Lift one arm and the opposite leg, keeping your forehead on the ground and your tummy muscles pulled in. Alternate sides. Move slowly and with control. When this feels easy, move to lifting two arms while leaving your legs and head down. Then try both legs.

Then try both arms, both legs and your head/chest all as one unit. Think about arms and legs reaching in opposite directions so that your spine is lengthening as you lift it off the floor. Don't forget to move slowly!

Working Out

Working out stimulates the sympathetic nervous system, increases heart rate, increases breathing rate and makes you sweat. It is great for building muscle and staying fit. Suggestions are to do resistance training (also known as strength training, where muscles are put under tension against resistance for a specific length of time or number of sets) three times per week for 30–45 minutes in order to maintain the body's ability to produce hormones effectively, put on muscle mass (starting at age 40 the body loses a pound of muscle mass every year!), maintain bone density and stimulate metabolism.

Also, walking briskly for a good 20–40 minutes several times per week and/or climbing stairs for 10–20 minutes gives the body a cardiovascular workout. This will stimulate the heart and lungs and keep those pumps in the body working!

You can combine your strength and cardiovascular training into the same workout, also known as a circuit, which is a very efficient way to about getting the exercise your body needs.

Following are some exercises for the large muscle groups of the body. These can be incorporated into any type of workout and may be changed by adding variations, using small equipment, altering the tempo or altering the duration.

Having these few basic exercises as your foundation will allow you to work on more complicated exercises with ease as you will have a strong base to work from.

- Jumping jacks
  If doing a full jump isn't good for you, then you can do heel taps side to side. Start with a 40-second burst.

- Squats
  Stand with your feet shoulder width apart. Hinge at your hips and sit your bum backward as though you are sitting into a chair. Make sure that your spine is still long and you are looking forward. Arms can be across your chest or up by your ears.

  Start with 10–12 repetitions, focusing on form.

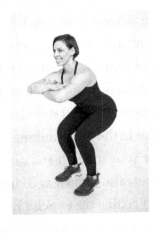

- Push-ups
  Start on your hands and knees. Make sure your hands are directly under your shoulders with elbows slightly bent.

  You can either come up onto your toes (as pictured) or stay on your knees. If on your knees, make sure that your hips are in front of the knees so that your body is at an angle. As you bend the elbows to come down into your push-up, lead with your chest. Hips follow along so that your bum doesn't end up in the air. Hold your tummy tight to ensure your back is supported.

Start with 10–12 repetitions, focusing on form.

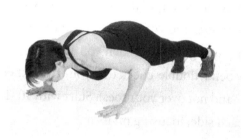

- Front planks

  Get into a position similar to your push-up position, but prop yourself on your elbows. Start on your knees. If you want to make it harder, come onto your toes (as pictured). You want a straight line from your ears, shoulders and hips to your knees (and your heels if on your toes). Aim to hold this position for 40 seconds.

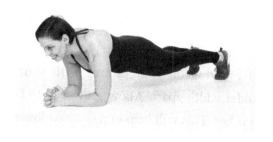

- Lunges
  Stand with your feet shoulder width apart. Imagine that you have skis on and you are going to slide one foot back within your ski track. Make your stride long, and ensure your feet are still shoulder width apart. Your toes should be tucked under with your heel lifted and your front foot flat on the floor. Bend both knees equally so that your body comes straight down the center. Aim for 90 degrees on both knees as your low depth (if that doesn't feel good, then stay higher up). When you are at the bottom of your knee bend, double-check that your front knee is over your heel (and not over your toes). Start with 10–12 repetitions for each side, focusing on form.

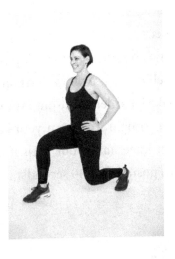

- Back extensions
  Start by lying on your tummy with your feet double shoulder width apart. Allow your heels to fall in toward each other. This will help to relax your lower back. Have your hands under your forehead. Think of reaching the

crown of your head, away from your toes, while lifting your head and chest off the floor in one piece. Your neck should still be long, and you should be looking down at the floor. You can choose either to bring your hands with you (as pictured) or to leave your hands on the floor for extra support.

Start with 10–12 repetitions, focusing on form.

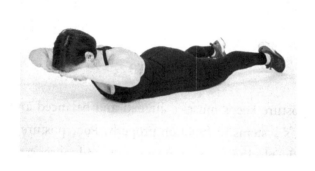

- Side planks

Lie on one side and bring your elbow under your shoulder, balancing on your forearm. Angle your hand forward. Start with your knees bent and your feet behind you so that you have a straight line from your ear, to your shoulder, to your hip, to your knees.

Another option is to have your legs straight, in which case your straight line will extend from hip to heels. Lift your ribs first as though someone has a hand under your waist, then lift your hips off the floor. Your top hand can be up in the air or on your top hip. Ensure that your shoulders and hips are stacked. Aim to hold the position for 40 seconds.

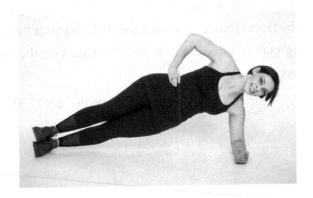

Posture

Good posture keeps muscles aligned and balanced and allows the body's systems to function properly. Poor posture impedes mobility by placing extra weight on joints and causes stress to the joints, muscles, tendons and ligaments, which can lead to pain. Also, the internal organs cannot function properly, blood flow is hampered and misalignments and disease may appear.

Remember that our muscles work as pumps to get fluids to move through our bodies. If a muscle is unbalanced or out of alignment, it cannot effectively pump. Poor posture almost always indicates a need for a stretching program.

Poor posture can come from not working a specific muscle enough or misusing muscles (poor technique or overuse).

Our muscles become either long and weak or short and tight like guitar strings. To tune a guitar, you have to loosen the tight strings and tighten the loose strings in order to play in harmony.

The same goes for the human body. We need to loosen the tight, shortened muscles and tighten the loose, weak muscles in order to have a body that is balanced and moves in proper harmony.

Therefore, it is important for us to stretch the muscles used during a workout, but also any muscles used on a daily basis during regular activities to maintain balance.

Foam Rolling

Foam rolling is stretching for the fascia. The fascia is the soft tissue that supports and protects most structures in the body, including the muscles. It covers all organs of the body, along with every muscle and every fiber within each muscle. Muscle and fascia cannot be separated from one another. The fascia goes from the top of the head to the tips of the toes completely uninterrupted.

We need to work on our fascia by rolling because the fascia can become irritated by trauma, surgical procedures, poor posture, overuse or inadequate rest between workouts. Fascia gets tight and knotted just like our muscles, but it doesn't stretch the same way a muscle does.

When irritation and inflammation occurs, it causes myofascial restrictions, decreases our range of motion and alters the motion of a joint. It can change the normal neural feedback to the central nervous system and therefore can cause pain. We then might have premature fatigue of a muscle, which can put us at risk for other injuries and cause us to have less-efficient motor skills.

Rolling causes gentle pressure to be applied to the myofascial connective tissue. Use a roll made out of foam, which causes an increase in blood flow to the area to stimulate your body's natural healing of that area. It releases restrictions and effects other body organs through the release of tension in the whole fascial system.

It feels like a deep-tissue massage, but you are in control of the pressure!

Benefits of Foam Rolling

- Corrects muscle imbalances
- Increases a joint's range of motion
- Decreases soreness and joint stress
- Maintains normal functional muscular length
- Breaks down scar tissue accumulation
- Removes lactic acid buildup

Tips for Myofascial Release

- Spend one to two minutes per muscle group on each side of the body (when applicable).
- When a trigger point (painful area) is found, hold for 30–45 seconds, breathing deeply.
- Keep the abdominal muscles tight, which provides stability when rolling.
- Remember to breathe slowly. It's not how hard you push but how deep you breathe that will release the fascia and muscle tension.
- Try to keep the muscles that are being addressed relaxed while you are rolling.
- After a manipulation, get up and walk around in order to encourage blood flow to the area.

- For best results, perform your rolling exercises before and after training, as well as within an hour and a half before bed. (If you don't have time to roll this much, then shorten your workout! Rolling is more important than lifting heavy things!)
- Use a tennis ball, a foam roller (which can be found at a sports stores or online shops) or a rolling pin.

Where to start? Most people don't stretch or roll enough. So if you are going to add anything into your life, it should be recovery and active release exercises. If you are feeling that you are not overstressed and are able to handle a workout, then resistance training is recommended. Next add in cardiovascular training.

Remember that you should never compromise your rolling and stretches for more workout time. In fact, as a rule of thumb, your warm-ups and cool-downs should match your workout time, for example, 15 minutes of warm-up (dynamic movements, rolling, gentle exercises to get you started), 30 minutes of working out, and 15 minutes of cool-down (foam rolling and stretching).

Stretching and Cool-Down

We need a certain level of flexibility in order for our bodies to function as they were meant to and for optimal movement patterns. Most people spend the majority of their days sitting (at work, at meals, in the car, in front of the computer or TV). If we don't move and stretch enough during the day, then we will have an overall decrease in flexibility and an increase in muscle imbalance. Eventually, things such as putting on your socks and shoes, and doing other everyday movements, will become difficult.

A lack of flexibility can cause injuries while doing simple everyday tasks such as vacuuming, making the bed or carrying groceries. Proper body mechanics can help these movements, but not if we don't have the proper range of motion.

You always want to do your static stretches when your body is warm. The best time is right after your workout. You can also do some gentle static stretches after a hot bath or shower. Static stretches are done while holding a specific position to the point of tension (but no pain should be felt!). Hold this stretch, remaining completely still with no bouncing around. Take deep breaths to allow oxygen to move into the muscles. This will allow your muscles to relax and stretch a little bit more.

All static stretches should be held for a minimum of 30 seconds with a two-minute maximum. Remember to do both sides of your body (even if only one side is tight or sore)! You don't want to be lopsided!

If you are doing a stretch with proper form and you are not feeling anything, then you probably don't need to do that stretch. Move on to another stretch for that muscle group, or move on to a completely different part of your body.

Here are some examples of stretches for the major muscles of the body. Hold each for a minimum of 30–60 seconds:

- Quadriceps (front of the thighs)
  Stand and hold one foot behind your bum. Slowly bring the leg in toward your body as far as you feel comfortable. Think about your thighs being parallel, and aim for your

knees to be together. Then press your hips slightly forward in space. Keep your chest up tall.

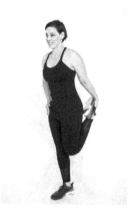

- Hamstrings (back of the thighs)
  Sit with one leg in front of you and the other tucked in. Sit tall and hinge forward at your hips, reaching toward your outstretched toes. Lengthen your spine.

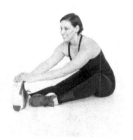

- Gastrocnemius (large calf muscle)
  Stand with one foot in front of the other. Bend your front knee and lean onto your front thigh. Slowly press your back heel into the floor. Adjust the back leg, moving it

either closer or farther away, until you feel a gentle stretch in your calf.

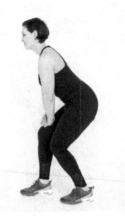

- Pectoralis (chest muscles)
  Stand next to a wall and bend your elbow, resting your forearm against the wall. Slowly turn your chest, tummy, hips and feet away from the wall. Stop whenever you feel a gentle stretch in the chest. Adjust the arm by moving it up or down the wall to a spot where you feel the most stretch.

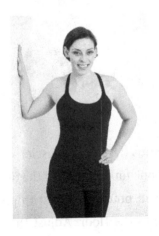

- Gluteus maximus (bum muscles)

  Lie on your back with your knees bent and your feet flat on the floor. Then cross one ankle over the opposite knee. Bring your bottom leg off the floor and toward your chest. Reach through your legs and hold onto the bottom leg with both hands.

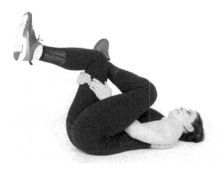

- Deltoids (shoulder muscles)

  Sit or stand. Put one arm straight out in front of your chest. Cross the arm over the chest and use the other hand to hold it in place. Lower your shoulders away from your ears.

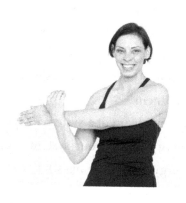

- Upper back opener
Sitting with your knees bent in front of you, wrap your arms under your thighs and hold your hands together. Pull your tummy muscles in and round your back away from your legs. Bring your chin toward your chest and allow your shoulder blades to separate.

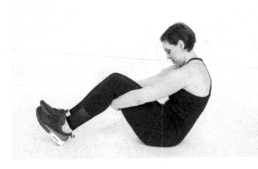

Working In

Working in is the opposite of working out. Working out exerts energy, whereas working in brings energy into the body. Working-in exercises do not increase heart rate or breathing rate. They stimulate the parasympathetic system. You should be able to do them comfortably on a full stomach (if you are working too hard, your digestion will feel compromised). These exercises will relax your mind and should never be so technical in nature that you need to think to do them.

The human body is made up of a system of systems. It takes energy to produce energy, and all our systems need energy to function (even the energy-producing ones!). For example, when you eat, you expend energy to digest your food. Your digested food produces the energy you need to be active.

Contraction of a muscle causes blood flow by the tightening and relaxing of the muscle. After the contraction, the muscle has to relax, which allows blood and energy to flow more quickly. The contraction has pushed the blood out of the muscle and into the veins to return it to the heart and lungs. When the muscle is relaxed, it receives reoxygenated blood.

So, the faster you move, the slower the energy flows in your body. The slower you move, the faster the energy flows. Therefore, all working-in exercises should be done very slowly and in a relaxed manner in order to help the energy flow. You will feel re-energized after you are done.

In fact, any exercise can become a working-in exercise just by changing the pace of movement. This includes breathing squats (squats done very slowly in time with your natural breathing pattern), a standing cross crawl (where you stand with feet shoulder width apart and arms in the air. Lift one knee and bring the opposite elbow to meet it. Return to starting position. Alternate sides), standing meditation, walking meditation, yoga, Pilates, tai chi and qigong.

Listening to your body is the most important thing. If you are under a lot of stress, then working out is not a good idea. Remember that physical stress is still a stress to the system. At these times, working in is the answer to regain energy and decrease stress.

Notes from Chapter 8

_____

_____

_____

Action steps:

    1)

    2)

    3)

    4)

    5)

CHAPTER 9

ENVIRONMENT

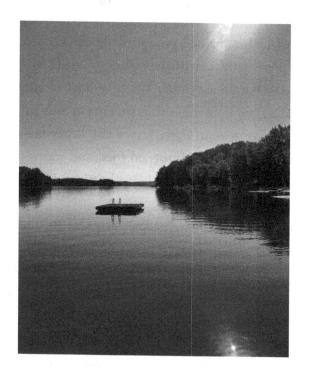

Many people don't realize how important the environment around them is to their health. Everything we ingest, breathe or absorb into our systems has to be dealt with by our filtration systems—and sometimes we can't handle it all! Remember that to be toxic means that we are taking in more toxins than we can get rid of. We can stop being so toxic by being aware of what we are surrounding ourselves with and what products we are using.

We have a very high-tech detoxification system built into us. Our lungs, skin, liver, kidneys and gastrointestinal tract all work to keep us toxin-free. If one of these systems is compromised, then we will have a hard time handling all the chemicals in our environment.

Sources of Toxins

Sources of toxins include processed foods, alcohol, caffeine, artificial preservatives, artificial colorings, artificial flavorings, medications, hormones, antibiotics (one dose of antibiotics or anesthetic can wipe out the healthy bacteria in your gut, allowing more infections in your digestive system), heavy metal toxicity from dental fillings, contaminated food and water, cigarettes, mercury, fluoride (which makes bones brittle and damages tooth enamel), lead and polluted air.

Air pollution kills more people each year than automobile accidents. The average person spends up to 90 percent of his or her time indoors. One source of pollution is the off-gases from carpets, pressboard, and glues that are used to build furniture. In fact, a commercially made piece of carpet will emit 130 toxic chemicals for the first year it's on the floor! Look specifically for environmentally safe products before bringing new items into your home. They are becoming more available in the stores, and companies are proud to be able to say they are being aware of our environment. So look for those products!

Microwaves emit electromagnetic pollution at a higher magnitude than any other appliance. Waves given off by a microwave alter the cells of our food to the point that the digestive system no longer recognizes it as food. The body then goes into an immune response, thinking that it has a foreign substance in it.

In a microwave, foods are heated from the inside out, which alters the atoms and molecules of the food and actually reverses the polarity of those atoms and molecules. We are physically hurting our food and making it not be food anymore! Start using your stove to reheat foods. It takes some getting used to, but eventually you won't even think about that microwave in your kitchen anymore!

Packaging is super important to look at. Any paper and plastics in packaging can actually migrate into our foods (especially when heated). Use glass, ceramic or stainless steel containers instead of plastic, and aim to be eating more whole foods and fewer packaged foods.

Water is a constant source of toxins—not only the water you drink but also the water you are exposed to daily. Your body absorbs 60 percent of what you put on it. There are about eight glasses of chlorine in a regular shower, so imagine how much you are getting into your system each time you shower. And water is not the only thing that is absorbed. Think also about beauty products that you use: creams, makeup, hair products, etc. Start reading labels. Just as with our foods, if you can't pronounce an ingredient, then you probably shouldn't be using it.

A new car emits over 60,000 toxic chemicals into its interior environment for at least the first year. When you sit in that car, you're literally ingesting those chemicals. Purchasing a second-hand car is the way to go! That way, you eliminate ingesting all those original "new car" smells and chemicals.

An easy way to tell if you are sensitive to environmental toxins is to gauge how you react to the smell of gas. If you feel nauseous or get a headache when near a gas station, it means that your immune system is too stressed to handle the toxins.

Go through your house room by room, along with any other space you frequent, including your office, and do a toxicity check. Look for items such as harmful cleaning supplies, plastic containers or dish ware, aerosol hairspray, air fresheners, hair coloring, vinyl shower curtains, microwave ovens, adhesives and artificial lighting. Add clean ventilation systems. Add filters to your taps and faucets. Replace as many items as you can with organic, environmentally friendly versions, or just throw things away!

Cleaning clutter also helps us to be able to clean more efficiently as less dirt and dust can settle where clutter is absent. Plus, we often feel lighter and freer when we declutter! So add regular clear-out sessions to your calendar. Whether it is with the season change, with the start or end of school, or just three or four random times throughout the year, booking it on your calendar will remind you that it's time to clear out your space and do a deep clean.

Here is an example of how to get started so that you can see the process without its being too overwhelming: Start by looking at one item in your home or office. Take paperwork for example. Maybe it doesn't feel toxic to have paper in your space, but an overabundance of paper certainly will take up space as part of your mind will be thinking about that stack of papers you need to deal with! Start by sorting into three piles: reference, to-do, and recycle. Each piece of paper needs to be dealt with and put into the right space. Next, dispose of the recycling! It will feel good to get rid of some things, and your space will instantly feel a shift in energy.

Then you should file all the reference papers in the appropriate places. If you don't have a system set up for this, do it now! Next, deal with those to-do papers. Pay bills, respond to clients, parents and school items, get things finished off, then recycle or file those pages as well.

Lastly, set up a system so that the paperwork doesn't get out of control again in the future.

This is just one example of how to start dealing with your environment. It can work the same for any item in your home or office, including furniture, artwork, toiletries and kitchen appliances!

Notes from Chapter 9

_____

_____

_____

Action steps:

   1)

   2)

   3)

   4)

   5)

CHAPTER 10

TIME MANAGEMENT

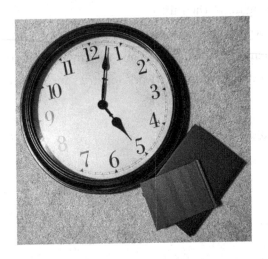

We have now gone over many ways to become healthier and live more holistic lives. But all of this can become overwhelming. How do we keep up? How do we manage our time in order to get everything done in the day and still have time to meal plan, meditate and foam roll before getting to bed on time?!

Let's look at different ways we can manage our time to be productive and still decrease our stress load.

1) Set up systems! Having systems doesn't need to be boring. You can still be spontaneous. But the systems will decrease

stress as everyone will know what to expect. Here are some examples:

If you have a predictable schedule, create a weekly chart to schedule everything in: meditation time, relaxation time, time to read or have a bath, time to do kids' activities (if you have to be there or just drop them off), time to work, etc. Start with the items that you do not have control over, then fill in the blanks with additional items. Make sure that you are taken care of as well. If you are going to be a good parent, you need some time for yourself and your partner! Create your own chart and fill in the blanks.

Now, even if you don't have a predictable schedule, or if your schedule switches all the time with shift work for instance, or if you are self-employed and your tasks change day to day, you can still create a schedule to help keep you organized and less stressed. If it's important, then it needs to be in your schedule. It may seem silly or unromantic to schedule quality time with your spouse, children or parents, but they should be number two in your life right after you! So if you book a business meeting into your schedule and turn off your cell phone and have no distractions, then don't your family members deserve the same consideration? Schedule the time and make it happen.

You may choose to use pocket notebooks with your to-do lists so you can add items or cross items off your list easily throughout the day. You won't have to keep all this information stored in your head anymore or feel the need to rely on an electronic device to store it. I highly suggest paper notebooks because then you won't waste time turning them on and having to find the right app—and you never risk the battery dying or not having Internet service. Make things easy and pop a notebook into your purse, pocket or briefcase before leaving the house!

2) Do some night-before planning. Now this may seem unnecessary to you, or you may be saying, "But I don't know what I have to do the next day until I get to work." Spend just five minutes each night thinking about how today went and what you didn't get done and/or what tasks you *have* to get done tomorrow. Write those down. This will allow you to stop thinking about all those items, subsequently relieving stress, calming your mind and allowing you to sleep more soundly. Then, when you wake up the next day, you can get to it right away without having to pause and figure things out.

It truly is amazing how much time we each waste by thinking about what to do next! If you have 10 minutes between appointments, for instance, you may spend five of those minutes thinking of what you can do that will take you only 10 minutes! Or you could have planned out those 10 minutes ahead of time to make them productive. Maybe that's your 10 minutes for breathing exercises or preparing for another meeting?!

3) Use large whiteboards/blackboards for charts, family activities, upcoming events, monthly to-do lists, etc.

Having items clearly displayed allows everyone involved to easily see what is coming up or what they are responsible for. It's pretty hard to ignore a huge whiteboard on your office wall or in your kitchen!

4) Make weekly item lists. This is a list or chart that identifies things you do only once per week but that happen each and every week. For instance, on Sundays you shop for groceries and do meal prep. On Mondays, you have 15 minutes of prepping for your week. On Tuesdays, you have 15 minutes of check-in time with your boss/staff. On Fridays you do a 15-minute cleanup of your desk so that it's neat on Monday to start your week fresh. Each week follows this same quick and simple routine. Without doing these tasks, you may feel that you are losing your sanity!

Notes from Chapter 10

_____

_____

_____

Action steps:

1)

2)

3)

4)

5)

AFTERWORD

Congratulations for making it through *The Pocket Guide to Mastering Your Holistic Health*! Now that you have read all the information, you may be feeling a bit overwhelmed by it all. Where do you start? I would suggest going back to your goal lists and taking a look at what you wrote down at the beginning of your journey. Are there things to add to your goal lists now that you have more knowledge of the human body and how it works?

Did you take notes and list your action steps at the end of each chapter? If so, go ahead and fill in your charts and your daily goal card with these new items. Start by focusing on achieving these goals each and every day so that they start to feel like a regular part of your daily routine and they become habits.

Next, look at your lists and which items you have marked as being the ones that are most important to you. That is where you go next. Take these important items and choose three to get going on right away. Remember that big goals achieve big things, but small baby steps will take you in the direction that you want to go.

Remember also that you are only human and that you will have the odd slip-up or experience times when you get distracted from your goals. That's all right. Give yourself permission to have your moments! You can go back and read any part of *The*

Pocket Guide to Mastering Your Holistic Health you feel necessary, keeping your goal lists and daily to-do lists close at hand.

Get right back on track as soon as you become aware that you have slipped. And don't get discouraged. It's when we make these tiny mistakes and then completely fall off the wagon that causes us trouble. But if you can pick yourself back up (and don't wait for a Monday or a New Year to do so!), you will be back to your routines and feeling healthy, happy and fit before you know it.

Now go out and get started!

ABOUT THE AUTHOR

As a child, Briar was diagnosed with Perthes disease, a degeneration of the bones, in her hip. Despite living with ongoing pain and repeated surgeries, Briar continued to train as a dancer and martial artist. She learned early on the importance of creating healthy, balanced practices for her mind and body in order to have the lifestyle that she wanted.

After completing her Personal Trainer and Lifestyle Coach Certificate, Briar began coaching her clients to do the same. Since then, she has worked with hundreds of clients and helped them level up and balance life, family and business while finding solutions to their health and wellness struggles.

Briar began working as a personal trainer in 1998 but wanted to create a better environment for her clients to reach their goals. In 2000, she opened Fly Girl Fitness, one of the top private gyms in the east Toronto area. Combining traditional personal training with her Pilates, dance, martial arts and mindset coaching background, Briar created programs that were unique and effective for her clients in a space that was comfortable and invigorating. Since closing her physical doors, Briar has worked virtually with clients from around the world to create that same atmosphere of positivity, safety and encouragement.

Living with Perthes disease, Briar knows that healthy exercise, nutrition and mindset is the difference between life in a wheelchair and life hiking through the woods with her two young children. These are the principles that inform her work with clients so they can be their best selves.

Check out *The Wellness Code*, the best-selling book Briar coauthored in 2012, and find her on Instagram and Facebook @ mindsetmamahealth.

Printed in the United States
By Bookmasters